AS I LIVE, DYING

AS I LIVE, DYING

VICTIMS OF WAR AND DISASTER

M.S. POWER

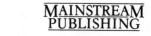
MAINSTREAM
PUBLISHING

EDINBURGH AND LONDON

First published in Great Britain in 1993 by
MAINSTREAM PUBLISHING COMPANY (EDINBURGH) LTD
7 Albany Street
Edinburgh EH1 3UG

ISBN 1 85158 502 8

A catalogue record for this book is available from the British Library

Typeset in Berkeley Old Style and Optima by Servis Filmsetting Ltd, Manchester

Printed in Great Britain by Butler & Tanner Ltd, Frome

FOR
LEX AND AUDREY CAIRNS

If only a man knew how to choose among what he calls his experiences that which is really his experience, and how to record the truth truly.

RALPH WALDO EMERSON

Contents

Acknowledgments

Clearly, because of its very nature and the demands it made on the privacy of a number of people, this book could not have been written without very considerable help. I would like to thank: Roderick J. Ørner, District Clinical Psychologist attached to the North Lincolnshire Health Authority, for allowing me access to his studies into PTSD, for his patience and generosity in advising and guiding me, and for tolerating with such good grace my many intrusive telephone calls and questions; Who Cares (Scotland) and Carolina House, Dundee, for their invaluable help in meeting young people who have suffered stress; Doug and Wendy Morris of the Gulf Families Crisis Line for their unstinting assistance in organising introductions which led to a number of the included military interviews, for the use of the material they had gathered, and for their unselfish willingness to share their findings; the Library staff of the *Scotsman* for their cheerfulness and diligence in seeking out the material I needed in such record time; and Joe McLeod of Dundee for his endless encouragement and the unlimited effort he put into researching many of the cases.

Above all I must thank those who agreed to speak to me, all those whose interviews I have included and those whose I did not. I am well aware that it took both great courage and generosity of spirit so to do, and my admiration for them knows no bounds. I hope they will feel that I have kept my word to them, giving their accounts fairly and without undue alteration, and that I have guarded their indentity as promised.

M. S. POWER,
DUMFRIES

Introduction

The condition known as Post Traumatic Stress Disorder – PTSD – has become one of the most discussed and, perhaps, one of the most misunderstood, medical problems in recent years. It was 'popularised' in the United States following the Vietnam War when many of the returning veterans showed behaviour that was inconsistent with their characters prior to the war, and was often inexplicable. In Britain, although the condition had been recognised after the Falklands Conflict, it was not until the termination of hostilities in the Gulf in 1991 and the return of the troops deployed there that it was accorded the same consideration as had been given it in America.

From a civilian standpoint PTSD has been diagnosed in people who had been involved in major disasters such as Lockerbie, the King's Cross Underground catastrophe, and the sinking of the Zeebrugge ferry. However, it would be wrong to presume that it takes involvement in *major* disasters to bring about post traumatic stress: a car crash, even the witnessing of same, can bring on the condition, and those in the services (police officers, ambulancemen and firemen) appear to be particularly susceptible.

Probably the earliest mention of what is now known as post traumatic stress was made by Samuel Pepys in his graphic account of both his own reactions and the reactions of others to the Great Fire of London in 1666. However, it was not until the nineteenth century that more formal appraisals of the psychological and physiological effects of massive trauma were made. American Civil War doctors observed 'states of physical and mental exhaustion', or neurasthenia, in soldiers involved in the fighting. A form of 'cardiac malady' has been mentioned in the official histories of the Crimean War, and included physical symptoms such as phobias, nightmares, and what was then described as 'chronic nervousness'. During the First World War the problem was called 'shellshock' and, as we now know, many cases were reported whereby soldiers suffered from anxiety attacks, insomnia and repetitive battle dreams.

Stresses, other than battle stress, gave rise to similar symptoms in the survivors of concentration camps and Hiroshima. Indeed, during the Second World War the experiences of the previous century led to the recognition that 'war stress' was a psychological trigger for all the variously named conditions: shellshock, battle neurosis and combat fatigue, to name but three. In general it was noted that these reactions, combined with feelings of emotional tension, cognitive impairment, physical complaints and, less frequently, conversion phenomenon, gave rise to the characteristics that are now sought in the diagnosis of PTSD.

As stated earlier, the Falklands Conflict renewed interest in the effects of trauma on the armed services in Britain, and while there appeared to be few cases initially, many instances of delayed onset were recorded subsequently. This may have been due, in part, to the reluctance of soldiers to report their condition to the authorities, supposing they recognised it, for fear of being thought of as a 'wimp' or of 'lacking moral fibre'. Northern Ireland, too, has produced a number of PTSD sufferers both in the military and in the civilian population. However, it is the Gulf War – the war, as many view it, that never happened – that has thrown up the largest proportion of cases. This is not to say that more servicemen suffered acute stress in the Gulf than in any other conflict; it means, simply, that the condition of post traumatic stress was more fully recognised following the Gulf War and consequently diagnosis of the condition increased.

And perhaps it is precisely because of its brevity, perhaps because there were so few dead on the Allied side, perhaps because it had received so much instant exposure on television that, in Britain at any rate, the possibility of survivors suffering from PTSD is regarded with considerable scepticism. In this context the military have come in for severe criticism often unfairly, in my opinion. They have been accused of 'closing ranks', of denying that PTSD exists in the armed services, of bullying and belittling those servicemen who report their suffering and seek medical help. It seems both injudicious and unwise to expect the military to know any more about this condition than the medical profession, and of the GPs I interviewed only 10 per cent had any real knowledge of what PTSD is. Some had never heard of it at all. Others gave a rather vague 'oh, yes' they had *heard* of it but that was all. Indeed, again in Britain, the whole question of the acceptance of the concept of a psychological response to stress continues to be controversial, even to the extent that some respected medics and health workers, like the criticised military, have expressed doubts as to the acceptability of such a disorder.

Post Traumatic Stress Disorder has been defined as the 'development of characteristic symptoms following a psychologically distressing event outside the range of usual human experience'. It is, at its simplest, a phenomenon resulting from intense fear, terror and helplessness, but it is singular insofar as one of the principal stumbling-blocks in recognising (and, hence, treating) the illness is that, in the vast majority of cases, the sufferer is unaware that he or she has a problem. Further, the general lack of expertise in both defining and diagnosing the problem has, inevitably, led to abuses. In the United States, for example, there has recently been a number of instances of alleged murderers claiming PTSD as the reason for their behaviour; and in Britain, compensation demands by people claiming to be suffering from the illness are on the increase. This has led to the curious and highly unsatisfactory situation where, too often, it is the *legal* profession rather than the *medical* profession which is being called upon to decide who is and who is not a victim of PTSD.

It is not, however, the province of this book to debate whether post traumatic stress is a disorder or a condition, nor is it intended to criticise what might appear to be the unwarranted diversity of opinion in the treatment of PTSD sufferers, nor to belittle those GPs who seem hopeful that the pills they administer will do the trick without even, apparently, considering the possibility that their patients might be suffering from something pills cannot cure. Having interviewed almost two hundred

15

people, military and civilian, who have either been diagnosed as suffering from PTSD or who have recognised by themselves that this is their problem, it has become evident to me that this insidious illness, whatever its definition, whatever its proper treatment, does exist, and that while the professionals bicker about the niceties very little is being done to solve the problem or to help the victims who are, as a general rule, left to cope as best they can.

In choosing which cases to include in this book I have tried to demonstrate the wide range of victims and to avoid the unnecessarily dramatic. One would expect Peter Grady, for example, to suffer from severe traumatic stress, but that Duncan Fosset should do so is perhaps rather less obvious. Yet there are many like him. I chose Duncan more on the basis of accessibility and his ability to put his emotions and feelings into words than for any more specific reason. Likewise, from both the Falklands Conflict and from Northern Ireland I had many examples to choose from: those discussed here are representative and the fact that they have been selected in no way diminishes either the plight or my respect for all the others who spoke to me.

One final point: it would be quite wrong to believe that post traumatic stress is suffered only by those who have been involved in or witnessed some major, well-publicised tragedy, although it is relatively easy to comprehend why they would. There are many, many people suffering equally severe stress but whose condition goes unrecognised simply because the cause of the stress is not fully appreciated. Unemployment over a long period, redundancy, failure by a student to pass a vital examination – the stresses of the modern age can cause trauma equal to involvement in war, a plane crash or a major traffic accident.

What had become clear, and common to all those whom I interviewed, is that they desperately seek some understanding and some help. Medical expertise apart, what most of them appear to crave is just someone to talk to, someone who will simply be prepared to listen – listen without judging, prescribing or criticising. For some sad and bewildering reason, possibly because of the current terminology used in defining the illness, stigma appears to be attached to it, and many victims refuse to seek medical help for fear of being diagnosed as mentally unstable and, possibly, being sent to some institution.

16

As will be seen, all those I have included and, indeed, every one I interviewed, are making valiant efforts to come to terms with their condition, and are simply trying to get on with their lives. Often they appear to be sadly fatalistic, accepting their current state and living with it. 'Just got to get on with it' is a phrase used over and over. It is also because of this stigma, real or imagined, that all of those who spoke to me requested that I conceal their identity, and this I have done. For that reason all names are fictitious, and most locations false.

In all cases I have allowed the victims to speak for themselves, interrupting as little as possible, and removing my questions from the transcript. It is a technique brilliantly used by Alan Parker, and I trust he will not mind my borrowing it.

ONE

Just one big cock-up, ain't it?

DUNCAN FOSSET

The voice on the end of the line was quiet, cheerful enough, with a West Country burr. This was the fifth time we had spoken, but we had written to each other many times over the last few months, and the hint of suspicion that had been clearly evident in his tone had all but gone. We had been put in touch by the Gulf Families Crisis Line, but I had only been given the name Colin.

Over the months I had explained the sort of book I was planning and had suggested that, if at all possible, it would make my task a lot easier if Colin could come up and stay with me in Scotland for a few days, where we could talk at our leisure. He had always agreed to come up, but had managed to find one excuse after another, but now he asked, 'Did you mean it about me coming up to stay?'

'Of course.'

'Okay. That's fine. I've been thinking about it and talking to a few of my mates and they said to go for it.'

'Right.'

'One thing: my name isn't Colin. It's Duncan. Duncan Fosset.'

'I see.'

'You don't mind my not telling you before?'

'No, I don't mind. You've got to be careful.'

'Yeah. Right. Well, about coming up. I can come just about any time. You just say when you want me and I'll be there. You know I'm attending the hospital now, don't you? I did tell you, didn't I? Well, I can get leave. Just you tell me when you want me up and I'll be up. I won't be able to stay too long though. A few days, okay?'

'Fine.'

He strode up the platform in Dumfries, swinging his suitcase. He was six foot two, blond, and looked older than his twenty years. Extraordinarily, he wore a wide-brimmed trilby. He was still several paces away when he smiled and held out his hand. 'See? I made it, sir.' His smile widened. 'Sorry about that. I know you hate it. Forgot about the "sir" thing.' He shook my hand, a surprisingly weak shake for such a big and clearly strong young man. 'Habit. In the Guards every bugger's a sir.'

That's your chair, I suppose? Yeah, thought so. Everyone has their own chair, don't they? Before he left us my dad had *his* chair. Nobody sat in it but him. Don't worry. I won't sit in yours either . . . It's different. Not what I expected. It's really nice, you know, and all, but not what I expected. Haven't seen an open fire for . . . don't know what I expected. You know you get this picture in your mind of somewhere? I think I thought it would be smaller and kind of dark. Can I look at the CDs? Hey, didn't think you'd have all these Pink Floyds. Well, you don't *sound* like someone who'd be into that. Not on the phone anyway. We can put one on later, can't we? Not now. Later. Great. You know the one 'The lunatic is on the grass'? Good that is. Really good.

Don't think I could live up here in a place like this. I mean, it's really nice and everything but it'd be too quiet for me. Like to have people around me. I mean, you could go weeks here without ever seeing anyone, couldn't you? Wouldn't like that. Would you mind if I take my shoes off? Don't usually wear shoes. Trainers mostly. Just put them on to be a bit sharp. Not really knowing what you're like, and all. That's better. Feel at home a bit now. Yeah, coffee would be great. You read all those books? There must be thousands. Don't read a lot myself. Sometimes I do, but not much. I've read some Stephen King. You read him? Good, he is. Really good. Got a bit more sugar? Just tell me where it is and I'll get it. Yours okay? Right, well then we can start talking if you want. No, no, that's all right. You can record it. I can listen to it later, can't I, and see what a wanker I am. No, I'm not bothered. Well, I am a bit. Not much though. The Crisis Line told me what you were doing and they say you're on the level so that's good enough for me. Not like those shitbags from the press. You've heard about them, I suppose? Gave my mum a bastard of a time. That was after – well after what I did, you know. So where do you want to start?

Okay. Right. Well, there's just my mum and my little brother and me at home now. And my mum's boyfriend. But family, there's just the three of us. We used to get on really well but now – since I got back – anyway, I'm jumping things. I always wanted to go into the army. Was in the Cadets and all, and was always watching war films. Don't know why it was. Just liked everything about it. So when I got into the Grenadier Guards I was pleased as fuck. Really made it, I had. Mind you, there was a lot of shit going on too. Bullying and crap like that but it's all part of the system, isn't it? And I mean if you can't take it, you shouldn't be in there, should you? I think the best thing was how proud my mum was of me. She had all these photos of me stuck up on the wall like a kind of altar. Mind you, I looked pretty shit cool in my dress uniform. Fancied myself, I did. So did the birds. Dead easy to pull them when they know you're in the Guards. Something really special, that is. You want to know all this? Okay. Well, if I start talking a load of crap that you don't want, just tell me. Don't want to give you crap, do I? No good to anyone. I could give you a load of crap and you wouldn't know I was doing it. But that'd be stupid, wouldn't it. Like fooling myself, really. I do that a lot when I'm drunk. You know about that, don't you? My drinking. That's a new thing too. Sure I used to drink, but nothing like I did when I got back from the Gulf. Think nothing of being pissed for a week. Vodka, mostly. My mum said I was becoming an alcoholic. Maybe I was, but I don't think so. Anyway, I've stopped that now. Nearly, anyway. Can't stop altogether, can I?

Anyway, I was stationed in Germany when the Gulf thing blew up. How did I feel about it? I don't know really. Haven't thought about that before. I think I was excited. We all were. Just kids most of us and we thought it would be a great giggle. We were hyped up quite a bit too. I suppose – I mean, I said I'd be honest with you – I suppose I was a bit scared too. Yeah, I know I was in the army and all that but it hadn't

21

really seemed like a possibility that there'd be a war – not a real war – when I joined up. Nobody'd thought about actually getting killed unless you were sent to Northern Ireland. So sometimes I'd feel a bit scared but you couldn't show that, so most of the time we were arsing around, letting on we didn't give a shit and that we'd really show that wop Saddam what proper soldiers could do. We pretty soon built ourselves up to a state where we couldn't wait to get out there. And the next thing we knew we were there.

Look, can I have a bath? I don't want to be cheeky or anything, you know, but I'd like to give it a rest for a bit. Thanks. Yeah. That's a good idea. Leave it till tomorrow. That's if it's okay with you. I can have a bit of a think during the night and I'll have it all sorted out for you in the morning.

Anything. I eat anything. Lasagne's fine. Maybe we can listen to some of your Pink Floyd later? Great. I'll have my bath now then. Don't go to no trouble now. Like I said, I'll eat anything. And I'll do the washing-up.

Not really. But don't worry about it. I never can sleep all that well in a strange bed. Anyway, gave me time to think, didn't it. You want to know something? I thought maybe I should forget the whole thing and go home. I don't like talking about it, you know. Then I thought maybe if I did talk about it to you – like, you're different to a doctor or a psychiatrist, aren't you – if I did talk about it to you it might do me some good. They tell you that a lot in the hospital – not to keep things bottled up inside you – but you know if you talk to *them* they're writing things down and trying to analyse everything, so you can't be really truthful in case you land yourself in the shit. I mean, I don't want to be locked up in some fucking madhouse, do I? You seen the TV programmes they done on those places? Jesus Christ! So anyway, in the hospital, we give them just enough to keep them happy and to make them think we're co-operating, but I don't think anyone ever tells them the whole truth. I shouldn't laugh, should I, but we have great laughs making things up. Like if it's a woman doctor we always talk a lot about sex and make up all sorts of crazy things, dreams and things, real erotic stuff, just to make them uncomfortable. There's one bloke in there and he should be a writer. Never known a better imagination. Mind you, he is in a bad way. Really fucked up in the head, he is. Don't think he'll ever get out. Oh, sorry, look, I didn't mean writers are fucked up. Okay. That's all right then. Didn't want you to think I hadn't any respect. I think that's important – respect. You think I'd be daft if I said self-respect was really important? Good. 'Cause I think it is. And that's sort of what I lost, I think. Self-respect. Maybe.

Anyway, there we were in the bloody Gulf. The first while was great though. Just like an adventure. We had all this special gear we had to get used to, and they gave us pills to take to protect us against germ warfare. No, chemical warfare. NAPS they were called. We were supposed to take – let's think a minute – can't remember – anyway we were supposed to take them at regular intervals but hardly anyone did. We'd wait until there was the rumour of a SCUD attack and then we'd just swallow a handful. We soon found out that by doing it that way we could get a good buzz, so it ended up that we'd do that – take a handful – if there was an attack or not. In the night time mostly, so our antics wouldn't be noticed. We used to call that the junkie watch.

I know you're waiting for me to tell you what happened that I think set me off, and I'm coming to that. Yeah, thanks, I'll take my time. No rush, eh? Am I allowed a drink? Just one. Thanks. I don't need it, you know. I'd just like one.

Okay. I'm ready. What way do you want to do this? You want me to tell you what happened when I got home first, or d'you want to know what I think it was that started the whole thing off? I'm easy. It's up to you. You're the one who's got to make sense of all this. Put it into shape. Suppose I tell you what went on in the Gulf now, and then later, maybe tomorrow, I'll feel more like telling you what went on when I got home. That be all right? Good. Cheers.

Well, the first thing you've got to understand is that all of us squaddies in the Gulf had been told we were in for one fucking hell of a war. The Mother of all Battles it was called. Now, most of us had never been outside England and hadn't a clue what to expect, so you can imagine we were pretty well psyched out. You know what that does to you? I'll tell you. What happens is all you talk about is killing the enemy. I mean, you build yourself up into a real state of hatred. And you don't just want to kill him. You want to cut him up. Cut his

23

bollocks off. We used to sit up and talk about what we'd do if we captured one of the bastards, and I can tell you what we said we'd do was pretty horrible. And it wasn't as if we were told to be calm or anything. Everyone was pleased we were getting ourselves worked up. One captain called it 'jolly good fighting spirit'. Stupid twat.

So now you're all ready, and then you wait and wait and wait. And what happens? Fuck all, really. Sure, we set off, thinking we were going to invade Iraq but we hadn't gone all that far before the war was over. I mean the fighting was over. Most of us felt really sick that we hadn't had a chance to fight, but we were all glad to still be alive. It might seem stupid or that I'm having you on when I say I don't really remember much of what we actually did, but I do remember one thing: we were heading towards Kuwait, following the tanks, and we came to this sort of ditch in the sand. It stretched out for miles. At the spot where the tanks crossed the ditch was filled with bodies. Dead Iraqis. I don't think they could just have fallen in there and piled up like that. More like they'd been stacked there like a kind of bridge. And that's what the tanks used them for. A bridge. Just rolling over them. Squashing them down. Made a fuck of a noise. Like someone mashing potatoes. Can't eat mashed potatoes any more now. Nobody said anything about it though. One bloke did laugh when I threw up, but nobody said anything. What? I don't know what they should have said. Should have said something, though. I know – this will sound daft – I know . . . well, you remember when I told you all the things we said we were going to do when or if we captured one of the Iraqis? About cutting him up and all? Well, here were some getting really cut up and all it did was make me feel sick. Hmm? No, not sorry exactly. I was glad they were dead, I think. But, well, I guess I was thinking we should show them a bit of respect because they were dead. It's different when you're dead, isn't it? I mean, you can hate someone as much as you like when they're alive, but when they're dead and can't do you no harm you should change a bit, I think, and show them respect. Anyway, that's the one thing I remember seeing and hearing. Naw, we never spoke about it after. Didn't want to seem soft, I suppose. Not good to show your feelings to your mates or they'll take the piss out of you. Can we stop now?

*

You hear me during the night? Good. I was afraid I'd wake you up. Oh, no, the bed's fine. Just couldn't sleep. That's why I came down and played music. I do that a lot at home. Play music during the night. I sleep better during the day when other people are moving about. No, don't worry, I'm fine. Really. I did have a bit of a kip in the chair. I had another drink too. D'you mind? Thanks. I sort of have this thing that if I'm asleep when everyone else is asleep and if I die nobody will find me until I'm gone mouldy. It happens, you know. People dying and not being found for weeks. Awful that. Anyway, that's what goes on in my head sometimes. I think maybe the quiet up here adds to it a bit. I mean, it really is quiet up here . . . Yeah, but only sometimes. It's a bit like I see myself – lying there all dead and squashed like they were. No, not squashed, just caved in like, and bursting at the sides. Sorry. No, you're the first one I've told that to. Couldn't tell them in the hospital, could I? Get myself locked up for good, I would. Anyway, they don't want to hear that sort of thing. Might make them have to ask questions or have an investigation and that's the last thing they want. You know what it is? They don't really want us to say there's anything wrong with us. Scared outsiders might find out and think the army's full of nutcases. Yeah, sure, I don't mind going back. Sorry for jumping ahead like that. I know it must be important to have everything in order. A beginning, a middle and an end, isn't that what they say? See, I do know a bit about writing. Where do you want me to go back to? When I got back? Okay.

Well, everything was okay while I was in Germany – that's where we'd been stationed and were sent back to. Just things started going wrong when we were given leave and I came home. I'll try and get this right but if you don't understand something or want me to explain something more, just stop me and say so. We've got to get this right, don't we? Well, to begin with you've got to know that I really love my mum and wouldn't do a thing to upset her. We always got on really great, like she was a mate more than a mum really. Sure, my little brother and me had our rows but we got on all right too. Maybe I gave him a thump when he nicked some of my clothes, but that was all. Nothing serious. So, anyway, the first thing I noticed when I got home was that they'd both changed. Now, I've been told since that it wasn't them who had changed but me. You understand that? But at the time

I definitely thought they had changed. I felt they were ganging up on me, trying to put me down all the time and wishing I hadn't come home at all. Now, don't ask me *why* I felt that. I mean, my mum still had all my photos up on the wall and I could see she was still very proud of me. And trying to think back – that's really hard, isn't it, thinking back and trying to be, what's the word? Yeah – objective. Anyway, trying to think back I can't put my finger on anything. You remember we were talking about that song 'The lunatic is on the grass'? Well, there's a bit in there that says something like 'there's someone inside my head but it's not me'. That's honestly what it was like. Is that crazy? And it wasn't just with family. I know that when I went out for a drink I'd find myself getting into fights – nothing serious, just punch-ups – for no real reason. And I had some money saved up so I bought this motorbike. Not new or anything, but a good one. No, wait a bit. *Before* I bought the bike something happened. I smashed up my little brother's room. No reason. Just smashed it up good. The thing is I *knew* I was doing it. No. I knew *someone* was doing it. It was me but it didn't feel like it was me. Am I making any sense? It was like this loony was smashing away and I was just standing there watching. What did I do after? Went out and got drunk, I think. Mum was really scared. I remember she kept asking me what the matter with me was, and telling me I'd changed a lot. That made it worse, I think because I kept telling myself – believing, really – that I was just the same and that they'd all changed. I said that before, didn't I? Anyway, it was after that that I bought the bike. I had it a couple of weeks when I smashed it up. Not on purpose or anything. Well, not really on purpose. I know I used to take a lot of chances and ride it dangerously, like I was trying to test myself or something. See how far I could go without killing myself, but I wasn't trying to do myself in, if you know what I mean. Anyway, the Vauxhall was bigger than my bike and that was the end of it. A complete bloody write-off. I went on a big piss-up after that. Lasted a few days . . . Yeah, let's do that. I could use a coffee. No, nothing to eat, thanks. Later. Okay? But you go ahead if you want.

No, that's all right. You can use all that. You can use anything I say. It's just when people say I said things that I didn't say that it pisses me off. Yes, I suppose I do sometimes but that's usually when they've given me some drug or something. Some sedation – that's when I might say things I don't remember. But I don't see the point of that. I mean if I'm not telling things about myself when I *know* I'm telling them it seems useless to me. I might be saying anything. And it can't be doing me any good, can it? The big thing they're always on about is the therapeutic value of opening up. But if you don't know you're opening up, where's the value in that, tell me? It's just a big cock-up, ain't it? Waste of time. Anyway, let's get on with this while I'm in the mood. While it's clear in my mind, I mean. Sometimes it isn't. Sometimes I can't think about it at all. Then, other times, like now, it's so clear it's like as if I can see myself doing it all over again. No, that's not right. I mean to say I can see *someone* doing it, someone who looks exactly like me, but me, I'm standing there in the background watching this moron making a fool of himself. I can even hear myself laughing at him sometimes. That's the crazy thing. Okay. Well, the best way to tell you about this is to tell you first what everyone says happened, and then I'll tell you what *I* remember happening. Would that be all right?

Well, my mum says that I came home in the afternoon and that I was in pretty good humour. I hadn't been drinking or anything. I'd just gone into town for a wander about. Oh, yes, I'd got a video to watch. Can't remember now what it was but if it's important you can phone my mum. She'll know. She remembers everything. You want to phone her? Okay. If it's not important. Anyway, she says I started watching the video and then after a few minutes I said I was tired and was going up to bed. About an hour later I came down – looking like a zombie, Mum said. I'd no clothes on but I said I was going out to a party. Mum's boyfriend was there, and my little brother, and I do remember that they all started laughing, thinking I was having them on, I suppose. I used to sometimes do daft things just for a laugh. I mean, pretend to be about to do something daft but not really intending to. You know what I mean? Acting the fool a bit. This time, though, they say I got really furious and took a carving knife from the kitchen drawer. No, wait. They saw that I did mean to go out in the nude and all and they tried to stop me. That was it. It was when they tried to stop me going out that I got the knife from the drawer. Now, the thing I can't understand is that it was my mum I grabbed and threatened with that knife. If I'd gone for my brother or Mum's boyfriend – well, it wouldn't have been

27

right but I'd understand it. But my mum. Like I told you I really loved my mum and would never have done anything to hurt her. But it was her I grabbed. I used her to get me over to the front door and then I ran out into the street. I can't help laughing at that now. Jesus, can you just see me running amok in this little village in the nude, waving this carving knife and screaming, 'come on you bastards'. Someone called the police. Not my mum. She called the Gulf Families Crisis Line who she'd been in touch with. Anyway, a couple of hours later they found me outside the village, sitting under some trees, crying. No, no. I hadn't hurt anyone. And that's what I'm told happened. Me? That's a bit muddled so you'll have to bear with me. Some things are very clear in my mind still. Like I remember being in my room – that must have been after I'd watched part of the video. And I remember getting undressed. I remember looking at myself for ages in the mirror. Not fancying myself. Just looking. I still had my Gulf combat uniform – you know, the camouflage one we all wore in the Gulf – and I think I remember taking that out and holding it up in front of me. I say I *think* I remember because I certainly did something with it because I was very proud of it and looked after it really well, keeping it pressed and hung up, but Mum found it all crumpled up in the corner of my room later. And another thing: I'm really very shy about being seen with no clothes on, so I think that when I went downstairs I must have thought I had that uniform on. I wouldn't – honestly I wouldn't – I wouldn't ever go about the house naked in front of my mum. So I must have thought I had some clothes on. Yes, I remember coming downstairs, and I remember them all laughing when they saw me. That didn't bother me. I thought they were – well, just laughing, and I was used to making people laugh with my daft pranks. I don't remember anything about saying I was off to a party. Nothing about that. I know I had to go out. I mean, I *had* to go out. I wouldn't want you to think I felt I had some – well, like some *mission* or anything, but it was . . . well, the truth is I thought the Iraqis were in the village. No, I thought they were coming into the village and I had to stop them. Not by myself, mind. My mates were all out there too, waiting for me to join them. I think that had a lot to do with why I threatened my mum with the knife. She didn't understand, you see, how important it was for me to get out there and stop the bastards taking over the village. And she didn't

28

understand that my mates would think I'd let them down if I didn't get out there to join them. Crazy, isn't it? You must think – well, no, you wouldn't. But you know something? I could really see the Iraqis. Okay, I've been told now that they were just the villagers and I imagined they were Iraqis, but at the time I knew they were Iraqis. And my mates had all gone. Don't know where. I think that's why I ended up well outside the village. Looking for them so they'd know I hadn't let them down. And I think I was crying because I hadn't been able to find them and I thought they would believe I *had* let them down. Oh, another thing I remember. I better explain first that the village – well, the house we live in – is on a bit of a hill and you can look down into the village proper. Well, I remember looking down once and there was this line of cars, just three or four but it looked longer, and I knew they were tanks.

After? When they found me? Like a right prick, that's how I felt. I mean, everything was back to normal. In my mind, like. And there I was bollock naked and crying like a baby and not really knowing what the fuck I was doing there. Sorry. I *knew* what I was doing there but I wasn't about to tell anyone, was I? Would you have told anyone if you'd thought you'd seen what I thought I'd seen?

Yeah. I feel okay. A bit stupid. I know you say you don't think I'm daft but you must think I am – a bit. Funny thing is, I felt great last night after I'd told you all about it, but this morning I feel stupid. You know, like after you've been drunk and done all sorts of crazy things that at the time seem like a hell of a lark but when you wake up with a hangover and get told what a moron you've been – a bit like that, I feel today. Mind you, it's easier talking to you, knowing I'm leaving tonight and don't have to face you every day. Don't get me wrong – it's been really good up here, but I'm glad to be getting away too. Yeah, back to the hospital. To be perfectly straight with you I think the hospital's a total waste of time. They keep talking about the PTSD thing but when you ask them what it is, no one seems to be able to tell you. And they're not *curing* me, like. I still keep having these – what are they – you know, they're dreams when you're awake – yeah, you could say that: hallucinations. I'll be walking down the street and suddenly, for no reason, it's not the street but the fucking desert. Oh, yeah, that was

29

another thing. I was up in the West End – we get weekend leave from the hospital, you know – and I was going to go to the cinema. There was this long queue and I thought, fuck that, I'm not queuing, and then the queue was those soldiers in the ditch I was telling you about. Just for a second or two but enough to make me feel like puking up all over again. No, I don't tell them in the hospital. Why? Why d'you think? I want to get out, that's why. If I keep telling them everything I'll be in there for the rest of my life, won't I? So I just keep saying, yeah, I'm fine, feeling really good today, slept really well, not a worry in the world. So I'm waiting to be discharged from the hospital and then I'll get my discharge from the army, and then – well, then we'll see what happens, won't we. I'll be okay, though. Bound to be. I can handle it. Getting used to it all now. So someone I know says, 'How are you?', and I say, 'Fine, great, couldn't be better.' Don't know what they expect me to say. Can't expect me to say I'm halfway round the fucking bend, can they? Maybe they do. But I sure as hell won't tell them that. And then maybe they say, 'Oh, you're better then, got over all that caper, have you?' And I say, 'Sure I am. I'm fine. Back to my old self. Just a bit of nerves it was, that's all. Nothing to worry about. I'm fine now.' And they believe me. So, you see, it's really only me that has the bother, and that's okay. No point in everyone else having bother. They can't *do* anything, so why bother them? Pointless, that is. Pointless. Makes them dead uneasy when I'm with them. Keep thinking I'm going to freak out, I suppose. Have another funny turn. That's what Mum called them – my funny turns. Yeah, some laugh *they* were. Laughed till I died. Someone said that, didn't they? Laughed till I died. What a way to go! But that's the way I feel about it. Huh? Oh, I mean, if it all gets too much, if I can't really handle it any more, I can always put a stop to it, can't I, one way or another? My option. Good having that option too. Like as if I didn't have that option I don't know what I'd do. Oh, yeah, I've thought about it. Not seriously though. Thought about it. Tucked it away back here as a possibility. Nearly said as a life-saver. That's a laugh. But it's a bit like that in reality. Knowing I *could* top myself if I wanted to helps. Helps a lot. Way out, isn't it? Escape route. Everyone needs one of those. What I'm saying is – look, take it I do go crazy again and really do harm someone, kill them maybe, well, there's no way they're going to lock me up in some nut-house for the rest of my life. No way, pal. So I use my option, don't I. Put a stop to everything there and then. A big round full stop . . . Yeah, you're right. I know it's easy to say all that sitting here. Maybe I wouldn't do it when the time came. Think I would, though. Why not? Better than being locked up. Much better. Just bang and I'm gone. Clean and easy. All they have to do is shove me in the ground and forget about me. Even me, I could forget about me. That'd be good. A relief, wouldn't it? Just lying there dead and not having to worry about something I might be about to do to someone. Yes, I think I'd like that.

Duncan Fosset was discharged from hospital in April 1992 and returned to his unit. In September 1992 he was discharged from the army for 'ceasing to fulfil Army medical standards'. Shortly after his return to civilian life he moved out of the family home and for several months did not contact his mother, although she heard he was living in a squat with a girlfriend. Duncan is now on remand in prison awaiting trial for breaking into a garage and robbing the attendant at knife-point.

TWO

I know what I'd like to happen

PETER GRADY

Peter Grady was in the same hospital, Woolwich, as Duncan Fosset and heard about me through him. While on leave one weekend he telephoned and volunteered to talk to me. He wouldn't, he said, come up to Scotland because 'my head's still mucked up and I do things at times that are a bit scary and I wouldn't want to do anything like that in your home'. We arranged an introductory meeting at a pub of his choice, about five minutes' walk from the hospital.

In contrast to Duncan, Peter was small, thin and wiry. His hair was dark brown and gelled. When he smiled, which was quite often, his eyes remained curiously opaque. His conversation came in hurried spurts interspersed with long silences during which he would just gaze at me which was, to say the least, unsettling. During our first meeting he smoked continuously, lighting one cigarette from another, and although we spoke for about two hours he only drank one pint of Guinness. He was very polite and was given to apologising frequently.

Sorry about this. I know it's not the best place to meet but I just thought for the first time it would do. Like, you mightn't want to talk to me again, and I mightn't want to talk to you again, so I thought this would be best. Neutral ground. If we don't get on we can walk away and no harm done, right? If everything goes well we can arrange somewhere better for the future. That's if we *do* meet again. We have to decide that today, don't we? I mean, what I have to say might not be any good to you. I don't really know what you want to hear. You might think it's all bullshit. And if you do, just tell me, and we'll leave it like that. Don't want to be wasting a lot of time or anything. But I'd like to talk to you if you can put up with it. There's not many people I can talk to. No family, you see. Haven't seen them for years. And I don't talk to my mates. Well, I have chatted to Duncan a bit but I haven't told him everything. He has his own problems and doesn't want to be loaded with mine, does he? . . . You're joking, aren't you? Nobody talks to the doctors. We don't want all this shit on our records, do we? Look at it this way – you get a medical discharge, what sort of a job are you going to get after that, tell me? Who's going to give a nut-case any sort of a job? Would you? So you keep your mouth shut and say, yes, much better thank you very much, and leave it at that. Let them decide from that. Yes, you're right. It would be better, I suppose, to talk it all out with someone, but you've got to find the right person. That's why I wanted to meet you. I thought maybe you'd be the right person. I mean, I'll probably never see you again once we're finished, so you're a stranger, and from that point of view it's almost like just talking to myself. Does that make sense? Good. I sometimes don't make sense, you know. I'm no good with words. I know what I want to say but can't find the words. And I do mean find. I *know* the words, they're somewhere in here in my head, but I can't find them, so I have to use other words that aren't really the right ones and then what comes out doesn't make sense. If that happens you've got to tell me. Will you promise to do that? I won't get upset or anything. If you're going to use what I say I don't want people to think I'm stupid. I'm not. I just get confused. So just tell me and I'll start again and keep saying it until I get it right. Like, we appreciate you talking to us and listening, so I certainly don't want to get everything all mucked up. I mean, if people – the ones who will read the book – if they *think* I'm gone in the head they won't pay much attention, will they? Yeah, Duncan told me you weren't going to change anything. Just write it like I tell you, so that's another reason for being careful. I hope you've got lots of time. That's all right then.

34

So what d'you think? Will I be any good to you? Yeah, I'm easy with you. Comfortable. Okay. Well, I get a weekend off in two weeks, would that suit? I don't want to give you the run-around or anything. Yes, I can meet you anywhere in London. No sweat. Sure I can meet at your publishers. Oh, it's a house. Even better, really. Can you put me up for the night if necessary? Well, that takes care of that. I'll see you in a couple of weeks. I'll phone you at home first, though. Just to make sure everything is still on. Yeah, you take care too. Nice meeting you.

This is nice. And they let you use it when you come down, do they? Must cost them a bomb just keeping this place for visitors. Oh, I see. It's their London office too. That's handy. Very nice it is. Must be plenty of money in books. Sorry – I don't want you to think I'm looking for a hand-out. I'm not. Really I'm not. Nothing like that. Anyway, I called you, didn't I? Not the other way round. Maybe I should be paying you. Just joking.

Right then. You want to make a start? Got that thing switched on? Right. Here goes. Don't forget now – if you don't get the point of what I'm saying just tell me. I won't mind. And something else I better warn you about. I might just dry up for a while and go all silent. Don't worry about that. Just leave me at it and wait. I'll come back to the point. I'm sorry about that but it does happen so I thought it would be better if you were prepared. Prepared for all emergencies, eh?

Well, you won't want to hear all about my childhood and crap like that. I'll just tell you I was born here in London. When my parents split up I was put into care. When I was old enough I joined the army. That'll be enough about that. It's got nothing to do with anything, really. Not with what you want to hear, anyway. Why did I join the army? Dunno. There wasn't anything else I could do, I suppose. I hadn't got an education as you'd call it, so there wasn't a lot of options. The army's full of blokes like that: soldiers because there wasn't anything much else they could do. Better than hanging about the streets and getting into trouble, isn't it? I mean, if I hadn't joined up I'd probably be in prison now. I'd started doing a bit of thieving, little things, stereos from cars and the like. Nothing serious.

Anyway, one day, there I was in the Royal Fusiliers. No, don't know why I went for them. Look at me. Couldn't very well get into the Guards, could I? Anyway, the Fusiliers it was, and I felt pretty good about it. Sure there was a lot of bullshit to put up with. There always is in the army. But I could easily put up with all that. No problem. And I felt I was doing something useful for once, and getting paid for it. And it was good to have mates. Never really had any mates before, you see. Not that I was what you'd call a loner. Well, yes, I was a loner but I didn't want to be. It wasn't by choice. Never really met anyone I wanted as a mate. We – me and my mates, I mean – were all about the same age – eighteen, nineteen – and we liked the same things. Music and everything. Having a bevvy. Chasing the birds. A disco now and again. You know they like to say the army's a family? Well, it's sort of true. My mates were a bit like a family. Brothers. Some of us got very close. We'd tell each other things that were really private. Intimate. Not the things you'd tell just anyone. I'll give you an example if you like? Right. Well, I was always worried my cock wasn't very big. So I told one of my mates this – after we'd been drinking, mind – I don't think I'd have had the nerve to tell him if I'd been completely sober. Anyway, he showed me his and his wasn't any bigger, so that really made me feel good. Got rid of a lot of complexes – that's the word, isn't it? Anyway, I'm telling you all this because I want you to understand just how really close we were. That way you'll understand why – well, how I felt when they were killed . . . Sorry about that. I did tell you I might shut up suddenly. Just thinking about it – even now, after all this time – it chokes me rotten. And it was worse for us, the one's that weren't killed, because of all the lying that went on afterwards. Sorry, jumping the gun, I am a bit. I'll go back. No, I want to go back. Think it through straight.

So, the Gulf War started and we were shipped out there. Dunno. Dunno how I felt. Can't rightly remember. Excited, I think. No, not scared. We didn't have time to be scared, it all happened so quickly. Anyway, we all kept each other cheery enough. Got to, don't you? One of my mates, one of the ones who ended up in *Warrior 23*, was always – look, sorry, I'm going to have to stop for a bit.

Thanks for having patience. No, everything's fine now. Just needed those few hours' break. It's pretty emotional stuff for me, and like I told

36

you I've thought about it a lot but haven't really spoken about it before. Not fully anyway. I'm going to try and do that but I can't promise it'll turn out like that. There's bits – I don't know how to put it – bits I can *see* in my mind but when I go to talk about them, something different – different words to the ones I want, I mean – come out. Like I'm not supposed to talk about them. Like they were my secret, although why I'd want them as a secret I don't know. Sorry. Yeah, okay, but it's not all right, is it? I said I'd tell you, and I want to tell you. That's the whole point in us meeting, isn't it?

You know what I think? I think it was a really sick joke to call it Friendly Fire. There was fuck-all friendly about it, I can tell you. What shithead thought up a name like that? Must be someone really sick, really perverted. Some wanker sitting behind a desk, I'll bet you. If he'd been out there with us he wouldn't have called it friendly. Sorry. I'm a bit paranoid about that, I know. Like they were trying to say my mates were killed in a friendly way, isn't it? I think so anyway. Making out it wasn't all that bad. Like they didn't understand that being dead is being dead, no matter what way it happens.

You want me to give you a bit of the background? Okay. No, I don't mind. That's the easy bit. You'll have heard most of it already, I expect.

The official stuff, anyway. That was all a pack of lies, you know. Everyone knows it was. You have to laugh, don't you, when you wonder how they thought they'd get away with it. I mean, did they think we were so fucking stupid we wouldn't know night from day? Oh, yes. Sorry. Well, it was Tuesday, January 26th. Me and the rest of the Company – C Company that is – C Company of the 3rd Regiment Royal Fusiliers, were pushing into Iraq. It was our very first day of fighting. There were thirty-seven Warrior Troop Carriers and support vehicles. We'd stopped to blow up some Iraqi gun emplacements. Not me personally, or those in the carrier with me. We were just sitting there in the back of the wagon doing nothing when this artillary started coming down on us. I think it was *Warrior 23* that got his first. I remember we tried to get out of the area, but it was all confused because we didn't know what the hell was going on. Then there was this other bang. Must have been *Warrior 22*. It just lifted up off the ground with the explosion. You know we hadn't had a single casualty and then suddenly, because of some American tosspot, there were nine of my mates dead. And you know what was really crazy? It was like it hadn't happened. I remember I just sat there on the ground beside my wagon and smoked a cigarette. Another of my mates took the time to have a shave. Someone else was reading a letter. Mad, eh? Just like we were all trying to fool ourselves into believing it hadn't happened at all. But knowing it had happened all right.

There's few things I've got to say here. Not that they've anything – I don't think they have, really – to do with my condition. But I want to say them if that's all right with you. Well, what really gets us – me and my other mates that survived – is the lies that went on afterwards. It was all political crap, you know, but it made us out to be liars when you think about it. Like the pilot of the A10 saying it was night and in the heat of battle with poor visibility. That was all bullshit. Like I've told you, it was daytime and we'd actually stopped to blow up those gun emplacements and there was nothing wrong with the visibility. Then he said he couldn't see our markings. Well, all I can say is he must have been blind or was lying through his teeth. All our vehicles carried friendly markings – a black V and then bits of fluorescent fablon taped on the top. Trev – the fleet sergeant in charge of seeing that those markings were on – always made sure they were on. And another thing, we kept those fluorescent strips as clean as a whistle – our fucking lives depended on them, didn't they? And another thing. That pilot said he thought we were T55 tanks. That's crap. Even a kid could tell the difference between a T55 tank and a lousy Warrior. That massive gun barrel on the T55 is a dead giveaway. The Warriors don't have them. And they're a dead different shape. And if that pilot couldn't make those distinctions at 8,000 feet – that's the height *he* said he was flying – he's nothing but a bloody liar.

Anyway, all that was bad enough, but when they held an enquiry – and that's a laugh in itself – it was like they believed everything the pilot said. So what did that make us? You tell me that. They really just wanted to hush the whole thing up so that the Allies wouldn't be embarrassed. We were told to say nothing, and for ages we didn't, but you can't let people go on lying, can you? It's not fair on the parents of

38

the lads who were killed for one thing, and it's certainly not fair on our dead brothers – that's what they were like: brothers. And I can tell you this for free – having to listen to all that official bullshit and keep the truth all bottled up inside didn't do my head any fucking good. I think, really, that did more damage than the actual killings. Well, it certainly added to it. If you get to talk to any of the other lads from C Company they'll tell you the same, I'm sure.

Okay. So you see what I'm like now, don't you? You wouldn't call me aggressive or anything, just sitting here having a chat with you, nice and friendly. Well, that's the way I always used to be. Never one for violence or anything. You wouldn't call me a psychopath now, would you? Not on what you know of me. But I'm supposed to be. I heard them talking about me in the hospital and that's what they have me down as, a walking psychopath. They think I'm liable to explode at any time. And I have to admit that on that point they could be right. I'll try and explain that because I think it's important. Before the Gulf and all that shit I was a great one for arguing. Nothing I liked better than having a good argument with someone, making my point and proving it. Now, though, that's all changed. First of all I've lost the ability to argue, and secondly I don't want to. I just want to kill any prat who differs with my opinion. And I'm not saying 'kill' the way you might say it – not meaning it. I *really* mean it, and I know it's only a matter of time before I do. Nice thought, that.

That's part of why I go off my head from time to time. That and the nightmares. Oh, sure, I have them all the time. Crazy ones. Like I'm in the desert and there's all these bits of bodies lying around like one big jigsaw and there's me, all alone, trying to put them back together. And it's all very frantic, like. There's a time limit on everything, and if I don't do it within the time, then my pals don't come back to life. Not ever. So, there's the nightmares, and there's this stupid feeling that I'm guilty in some way. Well, the way I see it is this: all the lads who got killed had parents and family. Well, I don't, like I told you, so why the hell wasn't it me that was killed instead of one of them?

Yeah, sure, I've told them in the hospital, but I don't think they know what I'm on about. I mean, they won't talk about it. Oh, sure, they want me to talk about it, but they won't. They just nod and say things like, 'I see', and 'what else'. Mind you, I was lucky. They all *expected* something to be wrong with me, so I didn't have to convince them none. But there's other lads out there who should be in hospital getting treatment and they're not. That's where your trouble is going to come from. Those lads will really explode sometime and Christ knows what they'll do . . . You're joking, aren't you? They can't do that. Not tell their officers. You want them to get lynched? No, the army's funny. Like I said it *is* a family, but it has all these rules, and the most important rule is you don't let the side down. You do that and you're shit. And going off your head is letting the side down. Letting it down badly. Yes, in the beginning a few lads did report what was happening to them and you know what they were told? Told not to be wimps, they were. Pull themselves together. Be men and stop being babies. Oh, sure, it's a bit better now. I mean the COs listen, but they still don't like it. Don't want to hear about it, and they sure as hell don't want anyone outside the army to hear about it. Damage the goddam image, wouldn't it. It's all right for other regiments to admit some blokes just couldn't take what they saw out there, but not theirs. You know what they'd really like? Just for us to forget anything even happened and just get on as before, just as if *nothing* had happened. That's why I carry these . . .

Look, I'm going to show you these. These photographs. You'll probably find them disgusting, but I seem to need them though I'm not sure why. Maybe it's because I need to *know* that someone else suffered and died besides my mates. Anyway, here – that's a pile of Iraqis dead after an air-strike. We came across them after we'd been hit. And that one, this is just one Iraqi soldier all burnt to bits. You can see the flesh peeling of him, can't you? This one's a bit of a laugh. We found these two curled up beside their T55. Dead they were, of course. So we sat them up and stuck a can of beer in their hands and had this photo took. That's me there on the right. Let's see . . . no, there's not much else. Just me doing daft things in the desert – having a pee and stuff – you don't want to see them. Well, okay, here you are, you can go through them.

Sounds weird that does. Me doing all that talking. Thanks for letting me hear it all again. No, you can use all that if it helps. Sorry about the language. You can cut that out if you like but it's the way I talk. No? Okay. Up to you. You're the boss.

Huh? That's like asking me what – I don't know what it's like. I've no idea what's going to happen to me. I know what I'd like to happen. This'll give you something to think about, I bet. Know what? I'd like there to be another war somewhere and I could go out there and really let loose. Do some real fighting – real killing I think is what I mean. Not this long-range stuff. That's shit. Hand-to-hand battle like it used to be. So you can see what's happening. That's what I want, if you want to know the real truth. Yeah, you're right, the excitement's part of it. The buzz, we call it. Ever had someone try to kill you? No, don't expect you did. But there's this buzz in that. Can't explain it. Gets every nerve in your body buzzing. Great. Weird too, but great. But I think too that if I could get stuck into another proper war it might get all this – this – yes, aggression out of me. It's all piled up and knotted inside me, see. It's all in here still, thumping about. All that aggression and hate. Got to get it out somehow, don't I, or just put a stop to it . . . You remember that bloke who went crazy in – where was it? – you know that small town – Hungerford, that's it, I remember now – that bloke who went off his head in Hungerford and shot all those people? Well, people kept asking why he did it, didn't they. Couldn't understand it at all, they couldn't. Well, mate, I *know* why he did it. I really do. Eh? No. No, I can't do that. I can't *explain* why he did it. I can *feel* it, though. I could be another one of those. Quite easily. Lots of us could. Could name you ten off the reel that could be like that bloke. It's a terrible thing to say, I suppose, and it really frightens me when I think about it seriously, but I think I need to kill before I can get rid of all the torment that's inside, and get back to normal. Ha, I *am* a psycho, ain't I? Must be, talking like that. Trouble is, I believe it's all true. Not saying it will happen. But it might, that's the point. It could. Easily. Doesn't even have to be an enemy. Just anyone would do, I think. Anyone. You maybe. That's a joke. No, not a joke really. That's what's so bad. I like you, see? But it wouldn't make any difference if it came down to it. Wouldn't think like that. Still, got to look on the bright side. Might not ever come to that. Could be another war, couldn't there? Looks like it, anyway. Let's hope there is, right?

41

The last I heard of Peter Grady was that he had left both the hospital and the army on a medical discharge, and gone to Bosnia to fight as a mercenary. I have been unable to verify this, although the information came from two different sources.

THREE

Yes, I still cry sometimes

CRAIG TOMKINS

Craig is thirty. He lives alone in a small council flat in Manchester. He has few possessions. The furniture in the flat is sparse, but everything is meticulously neat. The room we sit in is heated by a two-bar electric fire. Only one bar is on but the room still seems to be overheated. On a table beside his chair Craig has placed ten roll-up cigarettes – his ration for the day. He tends to smoke half a cigarette at a time, carefully extinguishing it, methodically saving the rest for later. 'That way I get twenty smokes,' he says. It is a very anonymous room: there is nothing to tell the visitor anything about the occupant – no pictures or posters, no ornaments, nothing to suggest he had lived there for nearly eight years. He might have just moved in. When he speaks his voice is very deep and quiet, and he gives the impression that he is a man who considers each word with care before uttering it.

Good of you to come all this way. I hope I'm not wasting your time. You'll know if I am or not pretty quick so you can tell me, and if you think I am, just you say so and we'll call it a day. I won't mind. Truly, I won't mind. I'll be sorry you had to come all this way for nothing, of course. But you won't hurt my feelings or anything like that.

Yes, that's right. It was all coincidences, really. My sister lives over in Coventry. She's been sick, so I went over to see her. If I hadn't gone I probably wouldn't have known you existed, let alone that you were doing a book on this PTSD thing. So, while I was over at my sister's I heard you talking to Maurice Dee on the radio. You were talking about the book you'd just written on child abuse, and then you mentioned you were about to do a book on sufferers of PTSD. So that's why I wrote to you via the radio station. After I'd written and posted the letter I began to regret I *had* written and, to tell you the truth, I sort of hoped either the letter would never reach you or that you wouldn't be interested. But then you wrote back so I had to follow up. I don't like messing people about. Life's hard enough without people messing you about unnecessarily, I think. But it seemed like such a good chance for me to talk everything out with someone that I had to take it. You don't mind? Like I said, if it's not what you want, just tell me. No need for apologies.

No. No. I've never actually been diagnosed as having PTSD. All I've done is read a lot about it and I'm intelligent enough to know that I probably am suffering from it. I'm not very intelligent, mind, but I'm not stupid either, so I could put all the supposed symptoms together and that way I could compare them to what was happening to me, and make my conclusion. Doctors? Not any more. I did when I first came back from the Falklands. Went to see my GP – that was in Coventry where I come from. He said I was probably just winding down and not to worry about it. He gave me some valium, I remember. Army doctors? You're joking. Of course not. At best they'd have said I was acting the baby, at worst they'd have given me a medical discharge, and God knows what they'd have put down as the reason for that discharge. It was like it is now since the Gulf. The Gulf lads are what I call the Glory Boys. They seem to be getting all the attention and, certainly, they're getting a lot more medical help than we did. We were just nothing when we got back from the Falklands. Oh, sure, the Paras got loads of praise, but us – well, nobody cared much about us. I suppose – this is just my opinion – I suppose with all the exposure the Gulf War got on the telly, people understood better just what war could really be like even though it was the poor bastard Iraqis who were getting the

44

hammering. During the Falklands they didn't show the really bad incidents, just the heroic bits, the bits that they knew people at home wanted to see. Stop them panicking. Stop them asking what the hell we were doing out there anyway. Oh, I know they give you all that business about defending British territory, us galloping to the rescue of the unfortunate Falklanders, showing the world that Britain could still look after its own – all that rubbish. But out there, out in that god-awful place, having to kill young Argentinian men and having our lads killed in return, we all wondered what in hell's name we were doing there. Not just us squaddies either. Officers too. They'd tell you the same thing if you could get them to tell you the truth. And I'll tell you something that really hurt. When it was all over and we'd got them back their islands, the islanders themselves didn't want us there. All they did was complain about everything we did. There was nothing victorious about it, I can tell you. They couldn't wait to see the back of us, and really didn't give a damn – or didn't seem to, anyway – that a lot of lads had been killed recapturing their stupid bit of land. Anyway, it's my opinion that the Falklands should be given back to Argentina, just like Northern Ireland should be given back to the Irish. It's just crazy hanging on to bits of the Empire in this day and age, don't you think?

. . . I can offer you tea. I don't have coffee. Don't drink it myself. But if you'd like some tea you're very welcome. Right. Just give me a minute.

Yes. You're quite right. Everyone I've spoken to thinks that – that there must have been one horrific, specific incident that affected me. And I'm sure it does happen that way in many cases. But not in mine, though. That's why I was worried I might be wasting your time. You see, I can't put my finger on any one thing and say that's what made me the way I am. It was just the whole combination of events. Everything from the mud and the rain and the cold and the fear and the business of having to kill. Yes. Of course. We knew we were soldiers and it was our business to kill the enemy if for no other reason than if we didn't kill him, he'd kill us. But you've got to understand we were all kids. Real *kids*. Even today, ten years on, the youngsters at the age we were then are far more adult than we were. Ten years makes a huge difference.

And although we were in the forces we never really thought we'd ever have to go to war. Like, in all our training it had never been suggested we *might* have to go to war. Apart from Northern Ireland, but even that wasn't looked upon as going to war. That was a peace-keeping operation, they said. So when war did come we were totally not prepared. What I mean by that is we were prepared insofar as we were trained how to kill, we had all the weaponry for killing, and physically we were really well equipped. But mentally I don't think any of us were ready for what was to happen. I honestly think that if the army had tried to get us mentally prepared they'd have had a mutiny on their hands. Well, I guess that's exaggerating, but a lot of the lads, me included, wouldn't have gone out there acting the gung-ho way we did. I have to wonder when I think about it: can you imagine all us young men going out there about to put our lives on the line and all we were doing was laughing and joking and thinking it was some sort of adventure, or an outing to Blackpool, for Christ's sake. There really was a sort of party atmosphere. Even on the QE2 that took us as far as the Bay of South Georgia, there were cabarets put on by the lads like we were on a cruise. Oh, sure, we were cramped, four to a cabin and all that, but I'm talking about the atmosphere that was being created, not about the physical side of things. It was the same on the *Canberra* that took us to the actual Falklands. The physical conditions were even worse on that. Packed like sardines, we were. But again, in the lounge, there were the cabarets with the bright lads showing how witty they were, or playing the piano and singing. All that sort of thing. So when it came to the crunch you can imagine what sort of shock reaction set in.

Did I tell you I was in the Scots Guards? I thought I did. Well, I can tell you that what came about on the Falklands was a far bloody cry from parading in Chelsea Barracks or guarding Buckingham Palace. In a daft way I think a lot of us believed because we were in the Guards and because we had these fancy uniforms that looked really smart, all we would ever have to do was *look* smart and parade ourselves for the tourists. Well, we soon learned different.

I'm not going to bore you with a minute description of the war, you'll know about that already, I guess. I'd like to try and give you images, if that's all right. The things that stick in my mind, the things that I believe have made me all messed up the way I am. The first image, and the one that really stays in my mind even though it's not frightening, is my first sight of the Falklands. All the way over everyone who knew anything about the place called it a right shit-hole, if you'll excuse that. They were right. They were being quite complimentary, in fact. We were hanging about, waiting for a landing craft to take us ashore, and I remember thinking who in their right mind would want to own a place like this let alone fight for it. Barren, treeless and grey. A place where on a good day it was just foggy, but where it actually just rained and rained and sometimes, for a laugh, I guess, threw in a few hailstones. It really was the sort of place they'd have sent murderers to serve their sentences in the old days.

Anyway, we got ashore eventually and started inland. Uphill. Everything seemed to be uphill. After about a two-hour slog the Company was placed in the usual all-round defence. It was time to dig in, but all that happened when you dug was that the water poured into the hole you made, and the deeper you dug the more water you had to cope with. As one mate put it, 'You'd need fucking webbed feet to live in a dump like this'. Everything was wet: our clothes, us, our equipment. Our boots were filled with water. It was the most miserable time you can think of. And we couldn't sleep because our sleeping-bags were filled with water too. A great start, wasn't it?

The next thing was the sicknesses. Nearly everyone got diarrhoea. The constant plodding about with water in our boots played havoc with our feet. I know this might sound pretty trivial to people but it was all part of the shock, you see, and it undermined, I think, the resistance we should have had to cope with the rest that was to come. Does that make sense? I'm just guessing at that.

Anyway, even all that misery didn't seem much more than a bloody nuisance. Yes, it *was* demoralising and all but it wasn't horrible. It wasn't exactly *war*, if you know what I mean. That came when we reached Tumbledown. That's when what we'd all thought war would be like really started . . . Well, even that's not quite true. All that most of us knew about war was what we'd seen on the telly or in films. And it's nothing like that. It's just one great big bloody mess, if you want to know. And I can't even say I'm haunted by the people I killed, because

I don't know if I killed any. I *shot* at them but whether I hit anyone or not I don't know. But I do know they killed plenty of us. That's the thing I am haunted by. Young lads having the life slivering out of them before my very eyes, and not a damn thing I could do about it but watch and cry for them. Yes, sure, I still cry sometimes when I think about it, and think about what it was all about. What was it all about, tell me? What did those young lads die for? Sweet nothing. Sorry. Yes, I still get really upset. Would you mind? I'll be better after a night's sleep. You got some hotel? I mean you can have my bed and I'll kip here, if you'd like. Oh, okay.

Fine. Fine, thanks. Your hotel all right? Good. That's good. Did you listen to all I said yesterday? Oh, was it okay? You sure? Good. I'm pleased about that. I thought, maybe, it was all – you know, I get confused about what I think is important and what other people find important.

So, I thought I'd tell you today what happened when I got back, if that's how you'd like it. I'm very clear about it all. I've been thinking about it for years, really. And especially after we contacted each other I've been going over and over it.

I think I knew just as soon as I got home that something was wrong. I don't say something wrong with *me*, you notice, because at that time I didn't know it was me who'd changed. Just noticed something wrong. I don't think I've mentioned that I was married. No, no, I didn't think so. Ha, I don't very often. Well, I was, with two kids. Girls. Both of them. Pretty little lasses they were – are still, I expect. No, I don't see them, any of them, any more. Better that way. For them. They're getting on with their lives. Karen, my ex-wife, she's getting married again soon. Had a letter from her via my sister. She used to write to me a lot to begin with but when I didn't answer, she stopped. Quite right too. Miss them? That's a hard one to answer. Can I put it this way: if things had been the same as they were before I went to the Falklands – when I got home, that is – then I know I'd miss them like hell now. But with things as they turned out, no, I don't miss them. It sounds terrible to say it but with me the way I am, they would be in the way. And all we'd do is fight and make life miserable for each other and the kids. No point in that. Much better I let her get on with things and me stay here by myself out of everyone's way. Here, alone by myself, I can control myself, you see, and if I do get mad at anything I can take it out on the wall or something. That way no one gets hurt but me.

Anyway, where was I? Yes. I got home and we were all given leave, of course. I phoned Karen as soon as we got back and told her when I'd be home, but for some reason, even then, I knew I didn't really want to go home. But I did. Had to, didn't I? Well, there was a litany of disasters. All my fault. Like you'd expect not having seen me for so long Karen expected we'd make love the first night, but I didn't. To tell the honest truth, I couldn't. Like I'd gone impotent or something. Just couldn't. Then I started drinking a lot. That was odd too since I'd never been all that interested in boozing just for the sake of boozing. Even when I was with my mates away from home, one or two pints was enough for me. But now I'd find myself going to the pub and staying there as long as it was open. I'd drink myself sick. Literally sick. And, of course, I was spending money hand over fist on drink, so Karen started in on me about that. Quite rightly. But I didn't see it like that at the time, so we had more rows. Then, one day, I just got in my car and took off. Don't ask me why. Karen said later that I phoned her from Plymouth and told her I wanted to be alone for a while, but I don't remember being in Plymouth or phoning her. I'm supposed to have told her too that I'd be home for the weekend, but I never showed up. When I did get back home I had to admit that I'd sold the car and spent the money on drink. Karen went bananas. I think it was partly about the car but mostly, *I* think, because we hadn't had sex at all since I got back from the Falklands and she thought I was having it off with someone else. Another blazing row, and what did I do? Took off again, didn't I. And that's the way it was for quite a while. But somehow I felt that if I could get away without having the pressure on me to go home I'd be all right, so I made up a story that I was being sent to Northern Ireland and would be away for a full tour. I was gone for about four months, I think, just living rough and drinking my head off. I'd phone home now and again, putting a hankie over the mouthpiece to make it sound far enough away to be Belfast. But in the end, of course, Karen found out. She was very good about it under the circumstances. Very civil. She asked me to come and just talk about it, and said that if we couldn't work things out I'd be free to do whatever I wanted. I

49

remember that's when I cried for the first time. Yes, I still cry sometimes. Not for any particular reason. I'll be sitting here nice and quiet and the tears will start. Anyway, we talked and everything I said seemed to come out wrong, or to be misinterpreted anyway. Like when I said I just didn't want sex, she thought I meant I didn't want it with *her*. When I said I felt she was a stranger, she thought I was *blaming* her. Anyway, the long and the short of it was that we broke up . . .

I don't know. I really don't know. I don't have nightmares or anything. I don't even think about the Falklands much any more except when something crops up on the telly. But something happened to me. It's like one part of my head isn't working any more. And it's like as if there's two of me: one person who's fine, like I am now, talking to you, being polite, I hope, and reasonable, and then there's this other person who takes over sometimes, who's violent and depressive and filled with crazy anger.

No, I don't bother about doctors much any more. I go along sometimes and get some valium or tamazapams and they help for a while. Drug me up. But most of the time I don't bother. Well, most of the time I just stay in here. Keeping out of the way. I don't want to harm anyone, you see, and I know I easily could if I go out. Just can't seem to control myself sometimes. Just go off my head and lash out. At anyone. Doesn't matter who it is. Doesn't even have to be someone who speaks to me. Could be that I feel someone is looking at me funny and in I go without asking any questions. Tell you what, though, sometimes it's like as if it's not really me at all. Like as if I was able to stand back and see this other person come out of me and cause the trouble. That's just stupid talk, I know. But it really is like that sometimes. Yes, I've been arrested. Hundreds of times. Well, quite a few times. Drunk and disorderly, mostly. Breach of the peace. Fighting. Brawling. All that sort of thing. Got to know me pretty well, they have, down at the nick. First-name terms with most of them down there. Get fed up with it, though, I do. That's why I try and stay in, in here, as much as possible. But I've got to get out sometimes, don't I?

No, I don't think I feel sorry for myself. I've accepted that my head's all done in. Just a fact of life. Anyway, there's plenty of others just like me as you probably know. Doesn't make it any easier knowing that, though. I suppose I do get angry sometimes that nothing was done, but then I think about it and I can see that they couldn't really have done anything even if they'd wanted to since they hadn't a clue what was wrong with us. Oh, sure, yes, they know *now*, or they say they do, but it's a bit late in the day for me, isn't it? Anyway, I don't want anyone messing with my head now. Too late. Make me worse, I think, if I let them start messing with my head at this stage. I've got things organised. I've organised the rest of my life and I'll just wait till I kick the bucket, and then it'll be over, won't it? That's it. It'll be over soon enough. Just got to wait. Do my best to keep things in check till the big day comes. Or night. Think I'll die at night. Don't know why. Always think that, though. Wait till the big night comes.

Two months after our interview, Craig was arrested for assaulting a police officer and causing actual bodily harm. He is currently serving a short prison sentence.

FOUR

We're cannibals, or didn't you know?

LES DIXON

His left arm is heavily tattooed. It is an intricate design of swirls surrounding the words 'QUEEN AND COUNTRY'.

The café is small. We are the only two in it apart from a woman behind the counter and a young man who appears from time to time from the kitchen. Les has chosen a table in the corner and sits with his back to the wall. He is in his late twenties, and sports a small, trim moustache. His eyes are very large and brown, and dart continuously towards the door and back to my face again. He places a packet of Regal Kingsize cigarettes on the table in front of him, and instantly starts to tear bits off the packet. His hands are remarkable, long tapering fingers with manicured nails. Hands more appropriate, one might have thought, to a surgeon or concert pianist rather than a Para. He notices me looking at them, and smiles. Clearly, he is used to people remarking on his hands.

Before I say anything you've got to promise you won't use my real name. That's essential. And another thing, if you use my stuff, once you've typed it up you destroy the tape. Don't want anyone recognising my voice. Got to protect myself. Still in the Paras, you see, and don't fancy getting a court-martial and being kicked out on my ass. Shouldn't be talking to you at all. Nearly wasn't going to turn up. And if you'd said the wrong thing when we met I'd have been gone faster than you could say shit. Anyway now we're here, I'm still wondering why I contacted you. Suppose because I need to talk to someone. Not an expert or crap like that. Someone who'll just listen and won't mind if I don't make too much sense . . . Yeah, I do realise that, but it won't matter to me if it's in a book as long as, like I told you – oh, hell, it doesn't matter, the name I gave you isn't mine anyway. Better you don't know. Better for me, that is. Got to think of number one sometimes. Be interesting to see my words printed up and know that no one knows it's me talking. Add a bit of mystery to it. Just you and me knowing and not another single soul in all the world. Tell me, what did you think when I rang you? Yeah, I suppose my getting your number like that was a surprise. Amazing how word gets round. People always talk. There were a few of us there when your name came up. One guy back from the Gulf had your number. Got it from the Crisis Line, he said. Know what? We were going to take the piss out of you. We were *all* going to phone you up and give you some story. Get you to come all the way down here and not meet you. Glad we didn't. You seem okay. Anyway, later in the evening I got that bloke to give me your number, and here we are, like I said. Lucky really I left it so long. I'm much better now than I was when I got back from the Falklands. Coming to terms with it, as they say. Coping. No way! Just by myself. *Couldn't* tell anyone. Been put down as a nut-case, and then where would I be? Out in civvy street with nowhere to go and nothing to do. That's why I'm being secretive about it. My life's in the Paras. If I had to leave I'd – well, it would be like losing my life. Don't want that, thank you very much. Let me loose from the Paras and Christ knows what I'd do, what would happen. Need my mates around me all the time. Know something? – this is the first time I've come out alone in – Jesus, I don't know how long. Always got one or two of my mates with me. Split for a bit if we pick up birds, sure, but when that's over, bang, we're back together again. Bonding, they call it. Very important that is, bonding. Helps. Helped in the Falklands, I can tell you. Never fight for yourself, you see. Always for the other guy, and he fights for you. Watches your back. You noticed? Yeah, I always try and sit with my back to the wall. Stupid, really. Just habit, I guess.

Sorry now I didn't arrange more time but like I told you this is just a quick meeting to size you up, to be honest. Yeah, you're okay as long as you keep your word to me. Think I'll be any use to you? Yes. Of course, stupid question. Have to wait and hear what I have to say first, don't you. Well, look, I can get the whole afternoon and evening off next Friday. Is that any good? Good. I'm sorry you have to drag yourself all this way down here again, but I had to be sure, didn't I? Anywhere you like. Why don't we meet here first, and then we can go somewhere more private if you like. Okay. Let's say – what time – two o'clock? Good. Two o'clock on Friday. You will come? Good. Yes, I believe you. Wouldn't waste my time with you if I didn't.

Hiya. Sorry I'm a bit late. Bet you thought I wasn't going to come at all. Had to wait on the tubes. Yes, let's do that. Better have something here first though, hadn't we. Then we can go to your hotel. Just coffee. No, nothing to eat, thanks. Maybe later. Maybe later we can go for a pizza or something.

All you need to know about my background is that I was born on a farm. My dad's still a farmer. Dairy mostly. I had an uncle who was in the Paras and ever since I was a boy that's what I wanted to be, a Para. And that's all I ever want to be and I don't want anyone mucking that up on me, you understand. I'm twenty-eight and single. Nearly got married once, but chickened out at the last minute. Couldn't stand the thought of being tied down. Didn't want the responsibility of a family either. I think if you're a Para that's all you can be. It's full-time. Nothing can get in the way. That's why so many marriages seem to break down with Paras. Wives don't understand – why should they? – so there goes the marriage. The regiment's our family. It's as simple as that.

When I was nineteen I joined up. The training wasn't that bad for me. I was pretty fit already. You try humping hay and straw around from the age of ten and you'll see how fit you can get. I was a good shot too, still am, come to that, 'cause I'd done a fair bit of shooting at home. In fact – and I don't want you to think I'm being big-headed or anything – the truth of the matter is that I was *so* fit and found the training *so* easy it got up a lot of noses. But the army, especially the

55

Paras, have a way of putting you in your place. Believe me, they do. And that's quite right too, I'm not complaining. You can't have individuals. It's a team, and it's got to work like a team. And once you're a Para, you're always a Para. Even if you live to be a hundred and ten you'll still be a Para. And think like one. Yes – I think so. I think we do have a special way of thinking. We're not brainwashed or anything like that. We just think differently to other people because of the job we're trained to do. Loyalty's very important, and I think that's a good thing. There's not much loyalty left in the world when you look around, is there? You see that series about the ex-Paras on the telly recently? You did? Well, I don't know what you thought about it but you remember there were letters in the papers and all saying it was all bullshit? Well, sure, there was a lot of crap in it, a lot of sentimental crap, but there were bits that were really close to the mark – like no matter how long you've been out the Paras, your Para mates come first. Always. I don't like using the word 'cause everyone takes it wrong, but we do love each other. I don't mean we go round kissing each other like they showed on the telly – that was really stupid, and embarrassing. And, anyway, what we feel for each other goes much deeper than that, but I don't have the words to explain it. It's just a feeling. A good feeling. Yes, sure we're tough. We're cannibals, or didn't you know? We eat our enemies. That's the myth. But it made us angry to see us portrayed as just mindless thugs always spoiling for a fight. I can tell you one thing: some of my mates are the gentlest men you'll ever meet when they need to be, but you never hear about that. It's what a reputation does to you, but our reputation is based on how we fight in a war situation. You know what it is? People don't look on *us* as people. That's what it is. We're sort of fighting machines and no one gives us credit for having emotions and feelings just like you or anyone else. That's why me and a few others have had to keep quiet about this stress business. Nobody would believe us. Machines don't suffer, you see, and like I said, we're supposed to be machines.

Sorry. You don't want to hear all that stuff. You can cut it out, can't you? Sure, use it if you like, but seriously, if you want to dump it, you just do that. Let's get back to what you want to know.

You ever been in a war situation? No. Okay. Well, it's going to be quite hard for you to understand then. Unless you've been there, under fire, you can't ever really understand. No one can, although you get a load of morons who say they do. They're just lying. It's like nothing else. I mean you can forget about all those grand things like patriotism and dying for your country and defending the realm. That's politicians talking. Look, think of it this way: supposing you, you as an individual, were being stalked by someone who wanted to murder you, okay? You and, say, your family, right? I can promise you the only thing in your mind would be to get the bastard before he gets you. You wouldn't be thinking about the morality of it or any of that crap. All that would be in your mind is surviving and protecting your family. Well, it's like that when we're at war, only on a bigger scale. There's hundreds, maybe even thousands of those bastards out there trying to kill me and my mates. So you block everything else out except getting him first and making sure it's them that get done first. You don't look on them as someone's son or father or husband. Not for a minute. They're just – just – just shit to be wiped up. That's all. And you've *got* to think like that. If you don't, if you start having the least bit of sympathy for them, you're dead, and some of your mates too probably, because you've always got to remember that they're thinking the same about you. That you're shit. The trick is to be cleverer shit than they are. Better trained. More dedicated. Maybe hating even more, although that's another thing. You can't let yourself hate *too* much because then you get blinded. It has to be a careful, cold hate. Controlled. That's it. *You've* got to be in control all the time. Let the enemy make the mistakes or drive him to make the mistakes, and then you've got him. Bang . . . Yes, you're right. It's when it's over and you have to come back to normality, as you say, that the trouble sometimes starts. But can I come to that in a minute? There something else I want to explain. D'you mind? I'd like just to get this out while I *am* talking to you. Thanks. Where was I? Yes. Going back to the guy who's out to kill you. Suppose you get to him first, right? You don't just kill him. I mean you don't just take one shot at him or stick the knife into him once. You make damn sure he's dead. You shoot him over and over or stab him several times. You want to make absolutely certain that he's never going to have the chance to menace you again. Part of the reason is that. Another part is the relief that you got to him first. And your relief, well, you might not like this, you might not even believe it, your relief makes killing him a kind of joy. You're actually *happy* to be killing him. Does that make sense to you? You're not agreeing just to please me, are you? I don't want that. Okay. Well, if you do understand that, you might be able to understand why things happen in war that afterwards are called outrages and stuff. Like they're saying now that some lads in the 3rd Battalion killed prisoners of war found hiding in the bottom of a trench after we – the Paras, I mean – had taken Mount Longdon. Now, I don't know if that's true or not – and even if I did I wouldn't tell you – but if it *is* true, it wouldn't surprise me. It's okay to be sitting nice and comfy behind a desk saying how terrible it is to kill prisoners, but out there, out there in all that shit, you're not thinking about conventions or things like that. What you're thinking is: here's a few bastards that as sure as hell aren't going to have the chance to kill me if I can help it. You're not saying, 'Oh, deary me. Sorry about all this. Do come along now like good chaps'. You're saying, more like, 'Fuck you Argie bastards for killing my mates'. I mean, you can't just switch on and off. That's what people expect us to do, but it can't be done that easy. Once you've psyched yourself up to kill, you can't de-psyche yourself at a moment's notice. Anyway, you don't *want* to. Put yourself in danger by doing that. Put the Company in danger. So, the way I see it is if a few prisoners were killed, well, that's just tough. They shouldn't have been there in the first place. And if the boot had been on the other foot, you can be pretty damn sure they'd have killed us. War is war, mate, and there ain't no niceties about it. I won't ask you if you can understand because I know it would be impossible for you, but try and think of what it would be like to have fought your way up a bloody Falklands mountain in all that rain and mud, with Argies shooting down on you and your mates getting hit and you expecting to get hit any minute. What state would you be in if you captured that mountain and found you were still in one piece? You're not in any state to be asking questions. You're still tuned in to the killing mode. So you come across these few Argies. Probably the same ones who've been making the last few hours hell for you. You're not going to sit down and discuss the situation with them. You're going to take them out. That's what you're trained for. That's what you're paid for, if you like. It's only when you get home, get some leave, start being sort of *normal* again that it all hits you. Yes, that's when it hits you. That's when – for the first time, really – that you might think about it . . . Ready for that pizza?

Handy that, just ringing down and having what you want sent up. Cheers. No, lager's fine. Don't drink spirits much. Now and again, but not much. Cheers. Ah, I could get used to this. Just kidding. Couldn't. Be an alky within a week. Go right to pieces. That's why I know it's important for me to stay in the Paras. Keeps me sane. Yeah, I know, people say the Paras aren't sane. Doesn't matter to us. They can say what they like. All we know is we're the ones they call on when there's some shitty job to be done. We're great lads then, all right. Anyway, I'm wasting your time. No? Jesus, you must get bored listening – how many have you spoken to now? That many. That'd drive me mad. I suppose that's true. If it's your job, you just do it. Can't see you lasting long in the Paras. Oh, sorry, didn't mean to be cheeky. Just meant it's not your job. That would drive *you* mad. Each to his own, I guess.

Well, then, yes, okay, like I said, it's when you get home and on some leave that you start thinking. That's what happened to me anyway. It started off by my having these nightmares. Real nightmares with me waking up in a cold sweat. And I could never shake them off even when I was awake and walking about. The worst thing was that I know I could have spoken about it all to my mates, one mate in particular, but I didn't want to. That was another part of it. I felt I'd lost something there. It was like I was looking at my mates differently. Like I didn't trust them. I *did* trust them – I'd trust them with my life, for God's sake – and I knew I trusted them but couldn't *make* myself trust them. Does that make any sense? The nightmares? Crazy stuff. Like I'd shoot this Argie, close range, and he'd fall down on his face and when I turned him over it'd be my dad or my older brother looking up at me. Or I'd be trying to kill an Argie and he just wouldn't die. I'd keep at him and at him, pumping bullets into him, kicking him, stomping on him and all he did was keep laughing up at me. Or – there was one when I was alone on this rise, looking down, and there'd be all these Argies coming up the hill at me. So I'd open fire. Mow them down. Watch them topple over. And when they were all dead I'd go down and it'd turn out that I'd wiped out my whole, entire own Company, and I could tell by their eyes that they knew it had been me who'd killed

59

them. Yeah, I know, I've found out since that that's pretty classic stuff, but I didn't know it at the time, did I?

Then there was the other thing. Like, I'm not a bad-looking bloke, am I, or so I've been told. I'm not a Frankenstein anyway. And I used to have a great way with the birds. I used to love the birds and really enjoy my sex. Suddenly that was all gone. Just didn't want to know. I mean, I wanted sex, everyone does, don't they, but something – no idea what – kept telling me I was dirty or something. Contaminated with something but I don't know and never did know what. So when the lads went out I used to have to make excuses. Stupid ones that I know they didn't believe. Oh, I don't know, don't remember – being tired was one, or I'd say I had letters to write – anything to avoid going out. And, of course, the more I stayed by myself the worse things got 'cause I'd all that time to think. I shouldn't have been thinking, brooding more like. And I started doing stupid things like getting my pay and going off and finding a room in a B and B and getting a load of booze and just spending the whole night drinking by myself. Yes, sure, I wasn't myself and could easily have fucked up but my mates guessed something was up and covered for me. No, they'd never do that. You don't with mates. Asking questions is like intruding. You do what you think best for your mate *without* intruding, but you're there if your mate wants you. That's the way it is. We respect each other's privacy. Okay, in my case it might have helped if someone had asked me what was up, but they didn't know that, and if I'd been one of them I'd have acted just the same.

Well, then I started this guilt trip. That's a real bitch. Drains you. Makes you want to curl up and – well, cry your bloody eyes out. But you don't want to cry. If you cry you're sort of admitting to yourself that you *are* guilty, and if you did that well, then, you might as well top yourself . . . About what? Everything. You name it, I felt guilty about it. About my mates who'd been killed. About the fact that they'd been killed and I hadn't. And the Argies became people and I felt guilty about them dying too. All crazy mixed-up stuff. I'd sit there in one of those B and Bs and go over and over and over my time in the Falklands and, you know what, I'd actually feel everything all over again, all the cold and the wet and all the noise. It was a bit like being in a trance, like, and when I'd come to, so to speak, I'd be freezing cold and the sweat would have made my body all wet like the rain had, and I'd have my hands over my ears to keep out the noise. Scary stuff, I can tell you. Yes, I did think I was going off my head, Guess I *was* off my head, wasn't I? . . . Can I use your loo?

Yep. Ten years. Ten years since the Falklands. A long time, isn't it, when you come to think of it . . . Well, let's put it this way: you've met me and we've spent some time together talking, how do you think I am? You really mean that? Good. That's very good. It means, doesn't it, that I've got myself under control? That's good. Well, you see, nothing much has changed except that I've learned to live with it. I still have the nightmares but maybe not as many. And I still haven't been able to have a proper, what I mean is steady, relationship with a girl. Longest any relationship has lasted has been – well, about two months. Then it breaks up. No, I always break it up. Even if I don't want to, I break it up. Hah, your guess is as good as mine. I just do, that's all. Feel crowded, I think. Like she – whatever girl it is at the time – is getting into my head, taking my space – and I don't want that. Can't take it. Need that bit for myself. Yes, sure it makes me feel lonely, but I can live with that. Got a bit of rank now and that helps. Makes me put on a good front so the men don't suspect anything. Makes me stop thinking too much as well. That's what it's about really – not thinking about it too much. Tuck it away and deal with it when you're on your tod. Won't cause any fracas then. Not to anyone else at any rate.

The guilt bit? Well, that's another matter. Another bloody kettle of fish. Yes, it's still there, but it's changed a bit. Let me ask you something – you religious? Okay, but you believe in God, don't you? And that when we die we go somewhere? We don't just rot away and give the worms a party? Right. I was brought up believing all that, but I stopped believing – no, that's not right – I don't think I ever stopped believing in it – you don't, can't, not once it's planted in your head. I just stopped thinking about it. Put it out of my head. It was easier like that. Made life easier if I did. Hard, difficult to be a soldier and have all that going on in your head. Well, I've started thinking about all that again, and you know what I think now? I think that when I die I'm going to come face to face with all the poor bastards I might have killed. That frightens the shit out of me. Not that I was wrong to kill them. It was war. It was my job. They'd have done for me if they'd had the chance. I just got in

61

there first and killed them. Still frightens the shit out of me, though, thinking I might come face to face with them. And in a weird way I've kind of told myself that if I do feel guilty for killing them they won't give me such a hard time of it when we meet. As if by feeling a bit guilty I was apologising. Not that that does them much good. Might do me some good though. That's how I think sometimes. Don't brood on it or anything. Don't think that. Just sometimes it crops up and I have a think about it. Anyway . . . got to get back. Better make a move. Thanks for everything. It's been good talking to you. Better than I thought it would be. Yes, you take care too. Just keep ticking along till the clock stops, eh? That's what we have to do. That's what I do. Just keep ticking along. All any of us can do.

And good luck with the book. Hope you have a bestseller. Can't see it though. Can't see people wanting to know too much about this stuff. Fuck them up. Sorry. Mess *their* heads up . . . No. No. You needn't do that. I'll keep an eye out for it and get it myself. Be funny to read all this in a book. Probably won't believe it all myself – that I actually sat down and told you all this. Really strange, that'll be. I suppose it will be like reading what someone *else* said, not me at all. But that's what it *is* like now that I think of it. There's me, and there's this other me. Maybe it's the other me doing all the talking. Better go before I really get myself confused. And you. Hey, you got a title for the book yet? 'As I live, dying'? Not bad that, mate. That's just about it. As I live, dying. A bit at a time. Cheers. Mind how you go.

A couple of weeks after the interview Les Dixon telephoned me to say thanks. He said just talking about everything had helped him get certain things (he did not specify which) into perspective. I was touched when he asked me to say a prayer for him. I have not heard from him since.

FIVE

I know *I didn't, but sometimes I think maybe I did*

ROBBIE FINDLAY

Robbie Findlay is twenty-two and has been out of the army for just over eighteen months. He lives with his mother and sister in a small terraced house not far from the centre of Dundee, and it is eleven months since he has stepped outside that house. He keeps himself fit by pumping iron in his bedroom. The only fresh air he gets is when he goes into the tiny back garden to play with his dog. For all that his complexion is good, his cheeks ruddy. He is a plump young man with bright red hair that he keeps cut only slightly longer than the style of a skinhead. His eyes are green and piercing. We have spoken many times on the telephone, but it has taken five months for him to decide to see me, and speak to me face to face. His accent is broad Dundonian which I will make no attempt to convey in writing.

Clearly he has been waiting for me and has the front door open before I get out of the taxi. His handshake is firm and he holds on to my hand longer than the norm, welcoming me and inviting me in, asking me if I'd trouble finding the house and how my trip up had been, before letting go. The sitting-room is immaculately clean and there is a smell of Pledge furniture polish. A bookcase runs the length of the wall under the window and is filled with videos. He indicates one of the armchairs for me to sit in, and settles himself in another, sitting forward, his hands resting on his knees. 'Just call me Robbie,' he says. 'No one calls me Robert.' He watches with interest as I test my recorder, smiling to himself. When I'm ready he runs both hands across his head and leans back. Immediately he is on his feet again and leaves the room, returning with a tray on which there is a pot of coffee and two mugs, sugar and a jug of milk. 'Nearly forgot. Mum would kill me if I'd forgotten my manners.'

I'm surprised you'd want to talk to me – you being Irish and all. That's why I was leery of meeting you. Didn't know who you might be. I'm like that now. Always thinking the worst. You hear stories, don't you? It's part of this whole thing. Part of the paranoia, I think. I'll be all right in a while. Just have to get myself settled. Don't meet strangers now. Don't talk to anyone outside Mum and Sheena. And myself. Talk to myself a lot. First sign of madness that, isn't it? Naw, don't think I'm *mad*. What's mad anyway? Just keep myself to myself. That keeps me . . . I nearly said 'safe' but that's not what I mean. Keeps me from being embarrassed. Stops people staring at me, or me thinking they're staring at me. That's more of it, me imagining too much. Those don't help, I think. Videos. Fill your head. Sometimes I'm not sure what's real and what I've been watching on one of those. But doesn't matter. Just myself to deal with. Doesn't harm anyone else. Look. Better tell you now. I smoke. No, I mean *smoke*. Joints. And I might need one. You sure? I can go out and – okay, then, if it's okay with you. That makes me feel better. Thought you might be, you know, very against that sort of thing. I call it my medicine. It really does help to keep me calmed down. I don't drink at all, you see. Never touch the stuff. Don't take pills either. Used to. Used to take them by the handful. All legal stuff, mind. From the doctor. Valium. Tamazapam. The usual. Found they weren't doing any good unless I took more than I was supposed to. Then found I was getting hooked on them. A pill freak. That frightened the shit out of me, so I stopped. So all I do is smoke a bit now. When I find myself getting jumpy. Had one just before you came. Tell the truth, if I hadn't I might have done a runner before you came. Naw. Never. I'd never bother with the hard stuff. That's for idiots. Don't need it anyway. Quite happy with a few joints a day. Been smoking for ages, mind you. Even when I was in the army. Often had a quick draw, we did, before we went out on patrol. Regular . . . That I don't know. Must have, I suppose, but they didn't do anything about it. Better to get us out there on patrol a bit stoned than not to get us out there at all. Don't think we were off our heads or anything. Nothing like that. Like, we had to keep our wits about us, didn't we, just in case. You never knew. Any patrol could have been your last. Sniper could easily pick us off. So it was just a couple of draws. One joint between three or four of us. Nothing heavy. But you don't want to hear all that. It's not important. Nothing to do with anything.

Oh, that was taken for granted. Was always going to be a soldier. My dad was a soldier. Dead now, he is. Car crash. Nothing to do with the army. And my grandad. Well, he was navy. My mum's dad, that is. My dad's dad was in the Royal Scots. So you see, I couldn't have done anything else. Wouldn't have been thought of. Don't think I'd have been able to do anything else anyway. Didn't want to do anything else either . . . No, can't say I do. I suppose if this hadn't happened to me I'd miss it all right. If I'd been kicked out or something then I'd probably miss it. But not now. Not the way I am. Took me ages to admit there was something wrong, though. Still don't know what *is* wrong. No, that's not true either. I know what's wrong with me. What I'm trying to say is I can't seem to make the connection between what's wrong with me and anything that might have made me this way. That's part of the reason I said I'd talk to you. Thought maybe you might have some ideas. Oh, aye, I understand that. I know you're not one of those psychiatrists. I wouldn't want you to be. Wouldn't have met you if you were. I just thought as we talked things might clear up a bit in my head, you know? I might say something, and then you might say something and between the two something might get cleared up. I'll never see you again after today, will I? It's pretty unlikely anyhow. So I won't have to worry about bumping into you and feeling like a right wanker because of something I might have said. That's good. Not like those therapy sessions they go in for where you have to keep going back and facing the same person week after week and him knowing all the crazy things you said the week before. That's not for me, I can tell you. No way. You can get yourself into serious trouble doing that, confiding in shrinks. Dead serious trouble. Like there was this woman up the street. Got depression fits and told her doc. Next thing she knew she was locked up in this psychiatric hospital like she was a fruit-cake or something.

Not for me, pal, thank you very much. Not for me at all. I'll handle my own self. And if it all ever gets too much there's always the big way out. Sometimes. Sure. Sometimes I've thought about topping myself. But not for quite a while now. When I was on those pills I used to think about it quite a lot. Just *think* about it, like. Never plan it or anything. Never even got round to thinking *how* I might do it if it came down to it. Just used to think there wasn't much point to anything if I had to go on drugging myself all the time . . . All right if I smoke now? What you mean? Oh, a cigarette. I thought for a minute – no, go ahead. Hang on, I'll get you an ashtray. Must be one somewhere. Maybe the kitchen. Hang on a tick. Oh, there. That there. You can use that. Put it there and we can both use it. Okay?

That's better. Aye, feel fine now. Ready for anything you throw at me. I'm doing a lot of talking, amn't I? Never thought I would. Not this much. I knew I'd have to say something to you after you coming all this way, but didn't think I'd be nattering on like I am. Already told you more than I've told most people. Uh-huh, I tried a couple of times. Ages ago. But you know what it's like. People don't really want to be bothered with other people's problems. Everyone's got their own and don't want another load of crap dumped on them. They don't listen when you talk to them. Didn't to me anyhows. Even my mum, you know. I mean, she pretends to listen but I know she's taking nothing on board. But you can understand that in a way. She doesn't want to think that there's something up with her son. So she just used to nod away and agree with me. Don't bother to try any more. No point. And if your mum won't listen, who's going to, answer me that? Aye, maybe, but like I said, the shrinks aren't for me. Anyway, I'm getting along okay now as you can see. I mean, I seem okay to you, don't I? Or do I? You think I'm acting okay? No, I'm not acting. I didn't mean it that way. No way am I putting on an act for you. I'm just being as I am. Honest. What'd be the point in agreeing to see you and then trying to fool you? No point at all. Dumb. It would be dumb. And I'm not stupid. Maybe I'm lots of things but I'm not stupid. Not saying I'm intelligent. Just that I'm not stupid. Funny that. As soon as something happens to you people think you're stupid. Gone stupid, just like that. I broke my leg once and was in hospital. That was years and years ago. When people came to see me – my mum and a couple of aunts, like – they never spoke to me at all. Know what they did? They'd talk *about* me across the bed like I was too stupid to answer for myself. A bit like I wasn't even there. Well, it's the same now. I know there's something not as it should be in here in my head but that doesn't mean I've gone crazy or anything. Am I making sense? I'll tell you for free what I really think: I think I'm doing pretty well even if I don't live like everyone else lives. Like I told you I never go out no more, but I don't think that's stupid. I think I'd be stupid if I did go out. That's what I think. Why don't I? Because . . . all right. I'll tell you. It's nothing to do with that sickness – don't know what it's called – a long name – that makes you unable to go out. Aye, that's it, I think. What did you say? Ag-o-ra-phobia. Yes. That sounds like it. Well, it's nothing to do with that. I could easily get up and walk out. Walk down the street or go anywhere I want. It's just that I don't *want* to go out. I'm coming to that. No, that's all right. Didn't mean to snap at you. Sorry. I don't want to go out because I know something will happen to set me off. Might be nothing you'd notice. A smell maybe. Or just seeing something, something very ordinary, that would remind me of something else, and then I'd start to panic, and Christ knows what I'd do. Example? Let me think a bit and I'll see if I can give you one . . . well, this isn't a good one, but once a car backfired and I thought it was a gun blasting at me. No. I've put that wrong. I *knew* it was a gun. That's the difference. You see, for me it *was* a gun. I didn't just think it was. Anyway, I really shit myself and my feet didn't touch the ground till I got home and inside the house again. But that's not a good one. Let's see. Funny. Now that I want to think of something I can't seem to. That happens a fair bit. Can't remember things or, like I told you already, didn't I, can't seem to see the difference between what really happens and what I imagine happens, or what I've seen on videos or telly. Aye, that'd be one. Shortly after I got out of the army I had to go down to the Bru for my cheque. I was walking along and there was this line of bins and plastic bags of rubbish waiting to be emptied. Then one of the bins just exploded. I saw it explode. I saw the flash of the flames and the smoke and I heard people screaming. That's what I saw and heard. But, like, the bin never exploded and nobody screamed, I don't think. The bin definitely didn't explode and yet I know I'd seen it go up. Sure as I can see you sitting

67

there now. Let's think what else. Aye. You'll maybe pack up and leave when I tell you this. No, I meant that as a joke. A funny. Okay, but you've got to understand that when I say I saw these things I really did see them. I mean *I* saw them. Okay, they weren't there but I *saw* them. All right? I can tell you the name of the street this happened on, even. Albert Street. Just a wee narrow street. Few shops and things. Flats. Some. Over the shops. I can't tell you why I was down there. Going somewhere else, I expect. And there was this blind man coming towards me with a cane. Tap, tap he went. Coming towards me. He was – dunno – a few yards away, ten, fifteen maybe – and he was a paramilitary with a gun. As simple as that. Balaclava, the lot. The next thing I know there's people pulling at me and kicking me and shouting at me. I'd only gone and attacked the poor sod, hadn't I? Knocked him to the ground and taken his cane off of him. Got done for that one, I did. They said I was drunk and I didn't argue even though I hadn't had a drink at all. Thought it better to let them think I'd drink taken than to try and explain everything. Got fined. Don't remember what. Not much . . . So there's examples for you, and that's why I don't go out no more. I'll make us another coffee, will I? You mind if it's instant? That's all we ever drink, even though mum fakes it up by putting it in a pot. Must tell you: she was dead nervous about you coming. Not about anything you might say to me. Don't think that. She knows you've had stuff on the telly and thinks you're Terry Wogan or something. Spent the whole morning yesterday cleaning this room out and tidying up. Then went over it again this morning before she went off to work. Back in a tick.

I knew you'd ask that and I was hoping you wouldn't. No. I didn't mean it like that. I don't mind your asking. Course not. Got to ask things you want to know, don't you? What I was trying to say is that I don't have the answer. I don't know why I'm the way I am. I've thought about it a lot, sure. I keep coming back to the same thing, the same one thing, but I'm not sure if that's why. Want me to tell you about that?

We was on patrol. Yes, Belfast. Just another patrol. Nothing out of the usual. I was plodding along minding my own business, as they say. Then, up the street there was a couple of shots and a lot of shouting. A kid had been shot. Not a *kid* kid. My age. My age like I was then.

When I got up there he was still alive, but he died pretty quick after that. I should, I guess, have been sorry for him, dying and all, but the truth is I was more worried about my mate who'd shot him. He was in a bad state. Shaking and all. Looking as if he was going to spew up. Anyway, there was an enquiry and all – there always is after someone's been shot – and it came out that the kid had a gun on him and that it'd been fired like my mate had said. That's not what's important. Now, look, I told you I'd been back down the street when all that happened. Fine. And I know I didn't shoot him. I couldn't have. But for some reason, in the days that came afterwards, like, I began to think that I had done it. I'd be doing something – anything – cleaning kit, having a game of cards, having a crap even – and I'd sort of see myself raising my rifle and shooting him. Even now, although I haven't thought about it much recently, I *know* I didn't but sometimes I think I did. Still. Mad, isn't it? . . . Tell who? Who was I going to tell? You don't tell anyone things like that. You keep that sort of thing to yourself. And there you are. That's the thing I think might have started all this. In fact, I know it started with that, but I don't know if it's the whole reason. What d'you think? No. Sorry. Shouldn't ask you that. How could you know?

It was lucky that we came back from Belfast pretty soon after the incident. Our tour was over. And we got leave. Change? Mum? Aye, well, she says now that she saw a change in me then. But you never know with Mum. She might just be saying that. I've never told her about – about what I just told you – but she says I was different. I've asked her what way I was different, but all she'll say is, 'Just different', which doesn't help a lot, does it? And Mum, anyway, is, I think, quite pleased with the way things have worked out. She likes having me here all the time. Ever since Dad got killed she's been scared of being left on her own. Sheena's engaged and is getting married in the summer. So she'll be gone. If I was okay I'd probably be thinking of getting married myself and moving out. That'd mean Mum would be on her own. She'd hate that. So she's quite pleased, you see, like I said.

Naw, I don't think about that at all now. Don't even have a girlfriend any more. No real chance of meeting one either. Much better that way. Couldn't really trust myself with a lassie, you see. And what if there were kiddies? If there were kids and I did something to one of

69

them? Not meaning to or anything. But suppose I did. No, better just to stay the way I am. And if I want the other I can always give myself a handshake. Sorry. Shouldn't have said that. No need for it. For me to say it. Sorry. Forgot myself a bit. Sorry.

The future? Haven't got one, have I? I mean, I never think about it so it doesn't exist in my book. The furthest I think is today. Just get through today and wait until tomorrow comes which, by the time it does come, will be today anyway, and then get through that as best I can. Maybe I'll click back to the way I was. Just like I clicked out of the way I was. You never know. Can only hope. That's all. Hope. But if I don't, well, then, I don't. No problem. I'll carry on just as I am. Going to be a few changes soon I think anyway. Mum keeps talking about moving when Sheena gets married. She's got this idea in her head about moving to the country. Even talks about going to one of the islands. Skye or Shetland. Maybe we'll do that. Can't really see it, but maybe we will. Could be nice that, couldn't it? Away from everyone. Maybe that's what Mum's thinking too. Getting away from everyone. Ah, well, probably still be here in twenty years, though. Wouldn't surprise me. Anyway, might as well be on an island here, really. Don't see anyone, and Mum keeps herself to herself, too, although she doesn't need to. We'll see. We'll see. Gas-pipe might explode and blow us all away. Never know, do you? No point in planning anything. Never know what's around the corner. Never know anything at all, really.

Some months later I was in Dundee and I called round to the Findlay house. It had new owners. I learned from neighbours that Robbie's sister, Sheena, had got married and now lived in Aberdeen. Mrs Findlay had sold the house and moved away with Robbie. Nobody knew where they had gone.

SIX

Something to do, isn't it?

DARREN KELLY

I had been warned that Darren might prove difficult. He had a reputation for making appointments and then not turning up; and being homeless, he was impossible to trace. I was also told to prepare myself for his violent changes of mood, swinging from the polite, beguiling and amusing to the abusive and threatening without a moment's notice or any indication.

At his request we had arranged to meet outside Boots Chemist in Piccadilly at 7pm. I was there five minutes before time and waited forty-five minutes. Darren never showed. At one o'clock in the morning he phoned me. He made no mention of our appointment but said he'd be outside Boots at eight that evening. He never showed up. And again, in the early hours he telephoned, this time saying he'd been busy but that he'd be outside Boots at seven. I agreed, but told him if he didn't arrive this time we had better abandon the interview as I had to get back home.

That evening he did arrive, bouncing up from the Underground. He was of medium height, and slim, with a mop of black unruly hair. As he crossed the road his limp was evident. I recognised him instantly from the description he'd given me and, clearly, he recognised me, coming straight up to me. He kept his hands in his anorak pockets and nodded. 'Hiya. Made it this time. What you want to do? Can we go get something t'eat?

71

I'm on a starvation diet. Haven't had nothing t'eat in a month. Oh, anything. Anything you want. Just food. Okay, whatever you say. You're paying. Let's move anyway. See them two pigs watching us? They're thinking you're some pervert trying to pick me up. Better move.'

I had been advised that Darren, to begin with, would probably exaggerate everything, and that I should take what he said with a pinch of salt, but that once he settled down and started to trust me he would tell me the truth.

Can't read this thing. What is it – Chinese? Well, can't read Italian either. Yeah – I can see it's in English underneath. I'm not blind. If you want to know, can't read much English either. I can do sums, though. Good at sums. You get something for me, will you. Yeah, steak is great. And chips. Can I have chips? No. No onions. No veg at all. Hate veg. Just steak and lots of chips. A Coke. Thanks. Me? Looking? Just looking. Like to look around, see what's going down. No. I'm okay. Just looking. Listen, you paying me something for this? Dunno. Something. Enough to get me into a hostel or a B and B for a couple of nights and a bit of grub. Yeah. That'll do. Whatever, have it your way. Call it helping me out. Call it anything you like just as long as you deliver. So, what you want me to say? You're paying, so tell me what you want me to say and I'll say it. What you mean – just talk? Don't get that. About me? Just talk about me? Okay, if that's what you want. I'll talk about me. Taking a chance, aren't you? Won't know if I'm telling the truth or just having you on, will you? I'm real good at making things up. Might be a writer myself one day. Got all these great stories in my head. Might write them. Make a few bob. Don't have to be able to read to write, do you? Wouldn't think so myself. Course I can write. Good enough.

Enjoyed that, I did. Best meal I've had in years. Belly's bursting. No, nothing more. Another Coke maybe. Don't drink coffee. Bad for you. All that stuff in it. Hypes you. You have one if you want. Hah, don't mention it.

How old are you? Don't look it. Not to me, you don't. Me? Twenty. Twenty-one in two months. Know I look more. Hard life, you see. Better to look older, I think. Over here, anyway. Less hassle. Don't get the perverts after you. Not unless you're looking for it. Loads of them here. Handy for the odd mugging when you've nothing. Suppose there are, but you don't see them much. Not in our part of Belfast. 'Fraid of getting shot, they are. Perverts.

Anyway, we're not here to talk about them, are we? Don't rightly understand what you *do* want to talk about. Yeah, I know you said about me. But what about me? Oh, that. Should have said. No, don't mind telling you. No big deal. Happens all the time. Part of the day. More Cassidys in Belfast than anywhere else in the world, they say. Hah. Cassidys. Hopalongs. Limpers. Get it? Good that.

You finished? Let's get out of here then. Getting closed in, I am. Getting – look, can we put off talking till tomorrow? Not pissing you around. Just want to leave it a bit. Okay, if you want to know – just wanted to see what you're like. Suss you out. That's all I wanted to do for now. No. Yes, I'll meet you tomorrow. Might get another feed, would I? Anyway, want to hear what I sound like on that thing. Be better tomorrow. Get my act together. My head . . . All the same to me where we go. Sure. Sure, if that's what you want. We can go back to where you're staying. Shepherd's Bush? I'll find it. Need a bit to get out there though. Just a bit. Needn't give me but the tube fare now. Got to deliver first. Never expect nothing unless I deliver. B and B? I can get one for about ten quid. But you don't have to. Okay. If you want. Ta. Yes. For sure. I'll be at Shepherd's Bush tube station at six. Six on the dot. See if I'm not.

Those oven chips were better even than last night's. Less greasy. Bad for you that is, grease. Makes the heart stop sudden. That's what I've heard anyway. Tell me, you keep that thing recording *all* the time? All the time? Why's that? Can't be much good talking about chips and stuff. That won't tell you nothing. 'Cept that I like chips. That mean something? Didn't think so. Up to you. Can I look at the telly later? Nothing that I know of. Just want to watch. Don't get much chance. Might be something good on. Never know, do you? Yeah, sure I miss the telly. Miss lots of things. Dunno . . . Everything. Pals. Mam and Dad. Home. My own room. You name it, I miss it. Doesn't do thinking about it, though. Go mad. Just got to get on with things till I can go home. Next year. Next June. That's what they said when they told me to get out. Make it a year in all. Not bad. Some don't get back for three

73

years. Some never. Could say I was lucky. Only a year. Just got to accept it. It's the way things are. Anyway, haven't got anything to cry about. I'd been warned. Twice, I think. Just brought it on myself. No point in crying now. My own fault. Yeah, sure. I can tell you about it if you want. Want me to? Okay. What you mean – background? Oh. That. Yes. Yeah, I can do all that. Like telling my life story a bit. Is that what you want? No problem in that. Easy peasy. Once upon a time, like.

Just the three of us: me, Mam, Dad. And the dog. Two cats, too. Dad? Nothing. Hasn't got a job. Been out of work over three years. Makes me laugh. Always at me to get out there and get a job, but can't find one himself, can he? No jobs going. Not unless you know the right people. Even then no guarantee. Doesn't really matter. Most people on the estate are unemployed. The way things are. Just got to grin and bear it. What, the joyriding? Let's think. Must have been fourteen. Maybe fifteen. Dunno. A while ago. Long time ago. Started with any old banger. The older the better. Easier to break into. When I was that age, I mean. Now, shit, five seconds and I'll get you into any car. Even the so-called burglar-proof ones. Tick-a-tick-a-tick and I'm in. No problem. Why? . . . Ever done it yourself? No, don't suppose you would. Well, if you haven't done it, you won't understand. Starts out as something to do. That's it. Something to do, isn't it? Gets rid of the boredom. Then, after, when you get into better cars and really start speeding, you start getting the buzz. Wow, it's a real buzz. Can't describe it. They say it's like drugs but I don't know. Don't take drugs. Not up to now, anyway. Like, I hear them all on the telly *calling* it a drug. S'pose it is. Can't stop, anyways. Got to get out there, behind the wheel. Yeah, sure, there's a bit of that. Everyone likes to show off a bit, don't they? I bet you do too in your own way. You want to prove yourself the best. So you drive faster and take more chances. Then that's not enough and you start taking the piss out of the pigs when they try chasing you. That's the gas. No chance with us. With me, anyway. I'm one of the best. Had about six of them after me one night. No chance. No chance at all. Had this Cosworth. Shit, could that baby move! Best night I ever had. Smashed it in the end, didn't I? Took this bend too fast. Skidded. Wham – into a parked van. Up in the frigging air I went. Landed on my side and skidded, dunno, a mile down the road. Bloody great, it was. But Vauxhall's is best. Dead safe, they are. Right nifty, too. Really shift.

Dead good on corners and brake-spins. Most I've ever got was three spins. Not stopping, I mean. Three spins, one after the other, in the same spin. You know what I mean? Not many can do that, I can tell you. Dangerous? Course it's dangerous. That's what's good about it. That's where the buzz is, knowing you might just kill yourself. Not that you think about that. You know you might but you don't think about it. Yes, sure, I know someone who was killed doing it. Happens. Died happy, I say. Stop us? Why? Don't care if I die that way. Better than spewing your guts up in some crappy hospital, isn't it? Got to go out with a bang. That's what I say. Who wants to live to be a hundred anyway? End up getting in everyone's way. Everyone just waiting for you to go. Not for me. Want to be dead and gone before I'm thirty. No hanging around. Okay. Okay. I take your point. All right for some. For you, maybe. But me – that's different. I've got nothing to look forward to, have I? No *prospects*, like they say. You think I do? You mean that? Never thought about having no death wish. Maybe you're right. Never thought about it. No. I know you're not saying I *have*. Don't think so. I'd do myself in if I had, wouldn't I?

Look, this is all crap, isn't it? Just a load of crap. I'm going. Forget it. I'm not saying any more. I'm off. See you.

Hello? Oh, good. You're still here. Thought you might have gone back home after last night. You want to see me more? Yeah. I want to. That's why I'm phoning. Yeah, I'm sure. Just got – you know. Doesn't matter. I can be round in minutes. Yeah. I know. Shepherd's Bush. That's where I am. Just cut across the Green, don't I? Yeah. I know. Be there in a tick.

They all as mad as me, these others you've spoken to? Bet not. Good to have someone different, isn't it? You like me? Don't get me wrong. Just, do you like me? Okay. I accept that. You don't know me. Don't know myself if it comes to that. But the bit you do know, you like me? You mean that? No. Doesn't matter if you do or not, but it's better if you do. Nice to be liked. I think I'm a likeable person. No. Like I said, I don't care if people *don't* like me, but it's handy if they do. Stops a lot of aggro . . . Okay. So, where do you want me to start now? Yeah. No problem.

75

Well, let's see. Better explain something about the situation first so you get the picture. Different to over here. Different to everywhere else, really. Take our estate. Police don't hardly come in there any more. Got our own law. Yes. That's right. IRA. Better than any pigs, if you ask me. No messing. Step out of line and you get it. Good thing is you *know* you'll get it, so if you do do anything stupid you've only yourself to blame. So, anyway, this time, a year back, the pigs started coming in 'cause we were nicking cars left, right and centre, and there'd been a couple of bad accidents, and a couple of kids had been badly knocked up. So we were told to cool it, or else. Came round to my house, they did. Two big fuckers. Frighten the shit out of you just to see them. Said I better leave off the joyriding. Start behaving myself like an adult. That's all they said. Did I stop? Hell, no. Got worse. Better it was, now that I knew I had to avoid them too. 'Course I knew they knew where I lived. Been there, hadn't they. But, like, I didn't think about that. Just wanted to show them I didn't give a toss for what they had to say. All of us did. Five or six of us that used to knock round together. They weren't going to shove us around. My dad was really scared. Kept on and on at me how I was going to get into real trouble. I mean *real* trouble. Even started locking me in my room. Soon stopped that, though, when he found I was just nipping out of the window, on to the porch roof and away. Even that made it all better. *Escaping.*

Yeah. That's right. Got another warning. Different blokes. Very polite and all. Spoke to my dad and mam first. Then hauled me down. Even told me what they'd have to do if I didn't stop. A beating, they said. Or maybe worse. They didn't say maybe worse, but you could tell that's what they meant. They don't mess about a lot. Yeah, I stopped for a while. About two weeks, I think it was. Then found I was getting all tensed up. My pals, too, they were the same. All strung out. Itching to have another go. It's the way it gets to you. *Got* to do it. Got to get into that car and drive like all hell was chasing you. Got to show just how good you are.

Too right, they did. I'd had my warnings, hadn't I? So this evening they came to the house. Not evening. Night. Real late when they guessed I'd be in bed. About four of them. Lifted me out of the bed and dumped me into their car. Couple of others had Mam and Dad in the front room, talking to them. Telling them not to interfere, I heard later. Drove me somewhere. Outside the estate. Kind of warehouse place, it was. Lot of timber lying about, I remember. You know, planks and things ready for selling. And they gave me a right going over. A *right* going over. Don't know what they used. Some sort of wooden bats. Baseball bats, like. Smashed one of my knees right up. Couple of ribs too. Four, I think. Christ, I was a right frigging mess . . . No. I'm all right. Use a Coke though, if you have any. Yeah. Lemonade'll do. Get dry, all this talking.

Okay. So, I spent a couple of weeks in the hospital. Fixed me up pretty good. 'Cept the knee. Couldn't ever get that right. That's why I've got this limp, if you've noticed. Told you I was a Cassidy, didn't I? Told you that one, eh? Good, eh? Anyway, did their best but couldn't do much. Great, they are in there. In that hospital. The way they can put bones back together would amaze you. Plenty of practice. But my knee – thing was just too smashed up to make a go of it. Fine now, though. No pain at all. Well, a little bit when it's wet. Wet seems to make it ache a bit. Nothing I can't handle, though. Just got to get on with it, don't you?

Yeah, I'm coming to that. Didn't like it much, all that delving into me. But that's the way they wanted it. After I started having the nightmares and stopped eating. That's when they started making me see this head doctor. Woman she was. Nice enough. Not pretty or anything. But nice. Nice to be with. Funny. I knew I was having the nightmares, of course, but never knew I'd stopped eating. They told me that I just refused to eat. Don't remember that at all. Can't have been hungry. You know what I'm like when it comes to food. Stuff myself. Not like me at all not to eat. But they say I just wouldn't. Didn't say 'I'm not going to eat' or anything. Just used to sit and stare at the food and make no attempt to eat it, and started going crazy when they tried to make me. No, not *make* me. Not force me. Just asking me to eat. Don't remember any of that. Started stopping people coming in to see me, too. No one. Used to take off for the piss-house if they came. That's something else I don't remember. All I do remember is I'd be in my bed at night and be thinking how glad I was no one had come in, even when they had come in and I'd done a runner. I wouldn't remember

77

them coming in, see. Wouldn't remember running off either. Just think they hadn't come in at all and be glad of that.

Yes. She explained it all. Had to go in for physio on my knee so she'd be there afterwards and we'd have these chats. Told me I was suffering from – dunno – shock or stress or something. Told her not to be daft, didn't I? Just laughed. Nicely. And started to explain that I mightn't know I was suffering from whatever it was – shock or stress. Didn't understand that at all. I mean, you'd have to know if you were suffering from those things, wouldn't you? Unless you were really off your head, which I wasn't. Anyway, she said I probably was, so I let her think that since it made her happy . . . That's enough for now, isn't it? Ta. Yes. You've guessed it. That's what I want. Got anything good? Oh. Okay. Let's do that. No. Don't like pizza. No Big Macs around here? There is? Let's go there, then. After that I'll toddle off. See you tomorrow, though, if you want. You want that? Okay. Give you a ring first. That's okay. Can't make it in the morning myself. Be same time as today probably, if that suits.

Stupid it was. I know that now. But couldn't help it, see? Nothing to do with the buzz I was telling you about, the one I used to get. That'd gone. You know what I think it was? I'll tell you. I think in some weird way I was trying to go back to before I got done in. Like something was telling me 'go out there and have you a gas and everything that happened will be wiped away. Wiped out'. Even took to driving up to one of the men who'd beaten me up. Slammed on the brakes so he'd hear me. And when I saw him looking out of the window, gave him two fingers, didn't I? Mad. Really mad. Looking for trouble. Yeah. That's it. Looking for trouble, I was. Like I wanted something to happen. Why would I want that? No, I don't know either. Maybe I thought they'd shoot me. Finish me off. Maybe that's what I wanted. Dunno. Just mad. Got to laugh though – me with this leg all in plaster, whizzing about like there was nothing wrong with me. Guess I wanted to show them they couldn't get me down. Maybe that was it. Dunno. That head doc – I think she knew, all right. Wouldn't tell me. Something about me having to find out for myself. Suggestion. That's a word she used a bit. Can't remember why. Oh, yes. She didn't want to suggest anything to me in case I latched on to it and used it instead of trying to find out the real truth. Stupid that. Didn't really want to know the real truth. Still don't, if you want to know. Think it might frighten me to death. Much better if I can just kid myself along.

Anyway, no, it was my dad who told me. Told me they'd been round and that I'd forty-eight hours to get the hell out. Do to me? If I didn't get out? What d'you think? No, maybe not kill me. But it would have been a worse battering than the other time and I wasn't hanging around to have that done to me, thank you very sodding much. Bad enough being a Cassidy without being a total cripple. Stuck in a wheelchair for the rest of my bloody life. Some life that'd be. No thanks. Don't make no turbo wheelchairs, do they? Getting pushed around all the time like an old man. Heh, get pushed around enough as it is without no sodding wheelchair. No thanks. Not for me at all.

So here I am like you find me. Yes, course I'll go home when I can. My home, isn't it? Where else would I go? No need to be afraid. Done my punishment by then, won't I? Just like being in prison, only – you know what I mean. Do your time and then it's over. Yeah, until the next time. Expect there will be. No, I don't. But could be. Always can be a next time. Habit mostly. Tell you one thing – they won't have to tell me to get out of there if there is a next time. I'll be gone. Won't see me for dust. Only happen if I lose control, though. I do that sometimes now. Lose control. Not sure what I'm doing. Do something and don't even remember doing it. Like it was a dream. Even, sometimes, have to ask, 'Did I do that?' Don't believe them half the time if they say yes. Don't believe anyone anymore, really. Not even myself. Great at lying to myself, I am. Can make myself believe anything I want even if I know it's a pack of lies. Really good at that, I am. Real talent for that. Helps too. Really helps, but you wouldn't understand that. Don't have to go round lying to yourself, do you? Pals? Here? Here in London? Naw. Not easy to have pals in London. Everyone too busy hustling to get by. No time for being pally. Always on the go, everyone is. Ducking and diving. A little bit of this and a little bit of that. You know – keeping yourself going against the odds. Anyway, like to keep myself to myself. In-de-pen-dent. That's me. Keeps me out of trouble. Don't have to know what someone else is up to. Just know what I'm up to. Not think about anyone else. Main thing is to keep on the move. Keep going. Lie down and I'll never get up. That's the way I feel, anyway. Lie down and

I'll never get up again. Don't want that. No thanks. Don't want that at all. Like giving in to everything, that'd be. Have to admit you couldn't handle it. Don't want to do that, do I? I'd really be finished if I did that. Just got to hang in there. That's what I say. I do what I got to do – as best I can, anyway. Hang in there.

That it? Oh. Yeah, I am a bit sorry it's over. Quite enjoyed that. Different anyway. Being able to tipple along without getting all sorts of shit thrown at me. Yeah, quite enjoyed that. Got what you want? Okay then. Say bye-bye then, I will. Yeah, bye-bye.

Before returning to Scotland I managed to get Darren a room in the home of two friends of mine who take in two or three homeless children and try to help them sort their lives out. On the second night of his stay, following a minor dispute about what to watch on television, Darren threatened another of the residents with a screwdriver. Admonished, he went up to his room. The next morning he had gone. Despite considerable efforts by both my friends and myself, it has proved impossible to trace him.

SEVEN

Grieving is just a way of life now

ARTHUR DUNLOP

Arthur Dunlop is a gynaecologist although it is now a number of years since he has practised. He is a tall, thin man in his early fifties, with thinning grey hair, and a stoop. He is very dapper and one of the most charming men one is likely to meet. His close friends are aware that he is homosexual, but there is nothing about his bearing or manner that would indicate this to the casual observer.

His home is a mews cottage, beautifully furnished. He has the largest collection of classical CDs I have ever come across. He has one oddity he admits to: music is played, quietly, night and day. This, he explains, is because he has found he needs music to calm him, and because he sleeps badly, catnapping throughout the day and night rather than resting for one long period. When he greets you at the door you feel immediately and sincerely welcome. 'Come in. Come in. How nice to meet you at last. Let me take your coat. We'll go in there, I think. A glass of sherry before lunch – yes? Just a cold lunch, I'm afraid. Cold salmon and salad. No. No trouble at all. A pleasure. I don't have that many visitors.'

It was so fortuitous. I hadn't wanted to go to that dinner party, but I ended up being persuaded. Friends, bless them, still trying to help after all this time. And I was seated next to our mutual friend, Helen. It was

81

over coffee that your book came up. We had been talking about the television, I think. Yes. That series you had on was mentioned. As being one of the highlights, I might add. Someone wondered if you were doing any more. It was then, I'm sure, that Helen told us of this book. Naturally, I was interested, and before we broke up I'd arranged for Helen to contact you on my behalf. The rest you know. Why? Why specifically? Well, and please don't think me arrogant, I was worried you might be being led to believe that this condition – PTSD – can only effect those who have been through some horrendous experience of a very public kind. You understand what I mean. War. Major air disasters. I wanted to try and explain to you that private tragedy can be just as devastating. I know that sounds terribly presumptuous – trying to teach you your job. You must forgive me if it seems that way. It wasn't intended, I assure you. But I know what the so-called experts are like. Not that I believe there are any experts in this particular field. Not yet, at any rate. So very little is known about it. I know of several mistakes that have been made – people diagnosed as suffering from post traumatic stress when their condition was equally attributable to some *physical* illness, and others who were not diagnosed who should have been. I'm afraid we're still at the stage when an aspirin is thought to be the cure where this sickness is concerned. In my own case, although I had a good idea what was the matter with me – inside knowledge, you might say – it was put down to mere depression, something I would get over as time went on. I was actually told that, you know. Time will cure. What a thoroughly stupid thing *that* is to say to anyone!

Anyway, let's have a spot of lunch and then we can settle down for a decent chat – if that's what would suit you? I've no idea how, exactly, you work, but I'll fit in, I hope, with whatever way you want to do this.

Yes. That's correct. But I wouldn't want you to think I latched on to it in any haphazard way. I mean, there had been quite a lot of talk about PTSD at the time. Particularly among my colleagues in the United States. And although it was well outside the realm of my particular practice we all knew something about it. It was a very slow, quite painful process but as the months passed I was able to be a little more objective about myself and diagnose my symptoms. No, no I don't blame anyone for not spotting it. I think it really comes down to the question of time. Effort also, but mostly time. I, you see, had all the time in the world. Contrary to popular belief, doctors do work very long and hard hours. They simply do not have the time to spend identifying, or attempting to identify, some illness that is not even generally recognised. But I had. I think, I'm certain in fact, that's the only reason I have been able to come to terms with everything. Knowing what's the matter with you is more than half the battle, you know. Once you identify it you can start doing something about it, which is what I did. Or tried to anyway. I'm not out of the mist yet, but I'm making headway. At least I can talk about it now, as you see, which is something positive. It's taken a long, long time, but that's how it is. How it should be, in fact. More damage is done, I believe by rushing the attempt at curing psychological problems than anyone can imagine. Time is vital.

Yes. Of course. No, I truly don't mind. If I thought I would mind I wouldn't have contacted you in the first place. Yes, I can understand why you might think that – that it would be difficult for me to talk about my very private life to a stranger, knowing that it might be published eventually. And no doubt *some* people will put two and two together and know it is me despite the false name, but I've come to terms with that. It really doesn't worry me. I've always been a very private person. Too private, I think sometimes . . . I can't quite answer that. It had nothing to do with shame, that I *do* know. I've never been ashamed of being gay. Confused as a young man, certainly, but, no, never ashamed. I didn't admit to it publicly for professional reasons. This may sound like an excuse but I don't offer it as one: I kept it to myself out of respect for my patients. Some women get very embarrassed about it. Some even wonder if a gay person can *be* a good doctor. Pregnancy can be a very nerve-wracking time for many women, particularly if it's their first pregnancy, and it was my duty, I think, to make as certain as possible that I put them at their ease, gave them confidence. Did what I could so that they would feel they could trust me, trust my judgment, trust what I told them. I didn't want to do anything to jeopardise that trust. And, of course, you must remember, we're going back a few years now when things were far less liberal, when the misconceptions about what gay people were like were unbelievable. But that's another matter – not what you want to hear about. You must make sure I stick to the point.

Indeed. Yes. But nothing that you might call serious. Very short-term relationships. The first one was when I was at college, I recall. Not that I was promiscuous – but don't think I say that to make myself sound in any way – what's the word? – superior, will that do? There simply wasn't a lot of opportunity in those days. One was extremely careful. One lived in dread of being thought of – well, as a sort of Quentin Crisp, if you understand what I mean. That sounds very disparaging to poor Mr Crisp. I don't mean it to be. He had, and always had, for that matter, far more courage than I'll ever have. Than many of us will ever have. I think what I'm trying to get across is that, all those years later, I was still somewhat naïve when I met Peter. That, I'm convinced, was part of the trouble. If I'd had more experience I wouldn't have become so obsessed. And it really was an obsession, you know. I'm aware of that now. A terrible, destroying obsession. But quite wonderful, too, in a dreadful way. It was a relationship that should never really have happened. We had nothing in common. Nothing to hold us together apart from my obsession. I was forty. Peter was twenty-four. He – if I tell you this, please, please don't think I'm being unkind – was barely educated, a bricklayer, no conversation. What they call 'rough trade', I guess. He was not even particularly good-looking. But there you are, I worshipped him. Simple as that. I worshipped him. No. No, we didn't live together. I, in a way, wanted us to, but it would have been very difficult to explain his presence. And in any case he didn't want to. He liked living with his family. A very close family in the – just off – the Old Kent Road. How long? I can tell you exactly: four years, eleven months and two days. It was eight days before his thirtieth birthday when he died . . . Yes, perhaps I will. Thank you. You're very considerate. I'll make some tea, I think. And perhaps change the music.

Indeed. Yes. That goes without saying. A total, complete and utter shock. I can't even begin to explain what it was like. You've heard the expression 'numbed with shock'? Well, truly, that is how I felt. Utterly numbed. Of course, now, in hindsight, I can see there were signs but at the time I never noticed them or, at least, misinterpreted them. Perhaps I just didn't want to admit they were there in case they disrupted our relationship. Looking back – and, God knows, I've done that often enough – I can recall that his moods, black moods, became more frequent. He could get very morose. No. I think not. Not depressed. Morose *is* the word. And introspective. Somehow you don't expect that in – well, in a bricklayer, do you? I know that's a terrible thing to say. Of course it can happen to just anyone, but you don't expect it in someone as *physically* strong as Peter was. Somehow, for no earthly reason, the physically strong are not really expected to be afflicted with any turbulence of the mind, are they? But, anyway, I had absolutely no inkling whatever that . . . Sorry.

I saw him on the Tuesday evening, and everything seemed perfectly all right with him. Indeed, I *think*, but I honestly cannot be certain, perhaps it's just *wishful* thinking, he was in one of the best humours he had been in for some time. I remember something had happened on the building site that had made him laugh. I can't remember what it was now, but he told me about it, and we laughed absurdly about it. We had a meal together. Here. Just the two of us. We watched some television. We spent a couple of hours in bed. I'd made a trifle for dinner. That was his favourite. His last words to me were that he'd be back the next evening to finish that damn trifle. He even warned me, grinning as he did, not to have 'a go at it myself'. But, the next morning, around four o'clock they said it was, he hanged himself in his bedroom.

Sorry. Even now. I am sorry. No, I'll be all right in a moment. There. That's better. I *am* sorry.

The biggest mistake I made, I believe, was to take a week off work. I should never have done that. I should have kept on seeing my patients instead of locking myself away here and brooding. That was quite disastrous. I'm sorry? Oh. As it happened, I couldn't see Peter as arranged. I telephoned his home to leave a message, and his mother told me. Mercifully she was so upset she just said he had killed himself and hung up. No, it wasn't as brutal as that sounds. As far as I can recall she said, 'I'm sorry. Peter died this morning.' I then asked her, I must have done, how it had happened. It was then she told me he had hanged himself. She wasn't being . . . she was just straightforward as

85

some people are. Oh, yes. She knew who I was. I mean, she knew me by my first name. I'd called Peter several times before. I was just one of his pals, as far as she was concerned. From the building site. No, I didn't go. I couldn't bring myself to go to the funeral, and I've had no contact with the family since, either. Two reasons, I think. One, because I was scared of, perhaps, the explanations I'd possibly have to make. You know how it is. His family, if they met me, would wonder what on earth Peter and I – you know. And second, in the most stupid way, totally illogical, I didn't want it confirmed that he was dead. Ridiculous, isn't it? If I'd gone to the funeral I would have been certain it was true, that it had, indeed, happened. But by not going, somehow I could convince myself that I still had a little hope to cling to, the hope that it was a mistake even though I knew full well there was no mistake. It was the emptiness, you see. The awful, unrelenting emptiness. And the guilt. You can't imagine the guilt I felt. Overwhelming. Absolutely soul-destroying. Of *course* I blamed myself for it, even to the point of considering killing myself so I could join him. I wanted to *explain* – I'd no idea what, since I really had nothing to explain. It was a dreadful period. Dreadful. Unreasonable though it was, that feeling of guilt persisted. And, as I said, the mistake I made – one of the many, I might add – was to take that break from work. Once I'd done that, you see, I'd capitulated. Given this insidious sickness its first hold on me, its first victory, if that's not being overdramatic. You see, in that week, that absurdly short seven days, doing nothing except grieving, the full chaotic web of the sickness had time to formulate. Mind you, I say I was grieving, and to a certain extent I was. But I would be less than honest if I didn't admit that I also was feeling very sorry for myself. Yet, to be fair to myself I think this was because I knew – oh, within a couple of days – that I would never be able to practise again. Why? You might well ask. I believe now that it was something to do with the fact that I couldn't face helping my patients bring children into the world in case they had to face – the children, I mean – in case they had to face either the awful sorrow that made Peter do what he did, or the pain which I was going through. That is melodramatic, I see that now. But at the time it seemed a perfectly logical reason for locking myself away. Indeed, it seemed totally proper and ethical behaviour. Convenient, of course. Most convenient, but I wasn't thinking like that.

You must, of course, understand that I was coming out of an *obsession*. I must stress that. Most people overcome bereavement as a matter of course and get on with their lives. I had done so myself when I lost my parents whom I loved dearly. This was quite different. An obsession, as I've said. And one of the factors about obsession is that, no matter what the odds – in this case the complete removal of the object of my obsession – you *never* let go. You are, bluntly, demented. And when, very slowly and painfully I had to admit to myself that Peter, in fact, was no more, things got worse. May I ask you – do you live alone? Ah. I'm sorry. You'll know then what it is like to suddenly find yourself isolated. How difficult it is – yet how imperative it is also – to make sure things don't slide. The mundane things. Eating properly. Shaving every day if that had been your habit. Dressing properly. Keeping yourself respectable. You have to push yourself to do all these things at times, don't you? Especially if you've nowhere particular to go, no one to meet. It's so very simple to become slovenly. Well, I became an utter sloven. Why I even bothered getting out of bed each day, I'll never know. But I would get up and then, still in my pyjamas, I'd come down here, sit down, and just spend the day staring at – at nothing. In the first three weeks I lost two stones. Just not eating. Picking sometimes but in an abstracted way. Habit more than intent. I never went out. Took the telephone off the hook. Never opened the front door. Oh, yes, certainly they did. Friends did call round to see what had become of me but I would tell them to go away through the closed door. I was abominably, unforgivably rude to them. Told them to leave me alone and to stop interfering. Why they – most of them, anyway – stuck by me is something I'll never know. Bless them. My partner in particular. He carried the full burden of the practice. I was just so *thoughtless*.

Oh, not for some time. Nor for several months. Only *then* did I start to recognise that something was wrong. Unbelievable, isn't it? All that time I didn't know anything was wrong with *me* apart from the fact that I was grieving for Peter. They say, I know now, that people suffering from PTSD simply don't know they have the condition. I would say that is true. Certainly, in my case it was. Most certainly.

Oh, Lord, I wish I knew. It might be of help to others if I knew. The best I can say is that it simply dawned on me that there was much more to my condition than simple grieving. I imagine my medical background helped. Of course it did. It allowed me to – let me say this – I agonised over the whole ethic of trauma. Can you bear with me a moment? Trauma, you see – and the Lord knows I've looked it up often enough – is defined as 'a morbid condition of body produced by wound or external violence' or, in psychological terms, 'emotional shock'. That's fine as far as it goes although it is, is it not, somewhat facile? But even accepting it as it stands leaves one with the problem of defining emotional shock. That is to say, what is emotionally shocking for one person need not be so for another. I think it is here that the whole question of diagnosis falls flat on its face. As you undoubtedly know by now, there is a standard list of symptoms of post traumatic stress by which the patient is assessed, and I do feel that, very often, patients are weighed one against the other – Tom had such and such symptoms and had PTSD; Bill has been through the same traumatic experience so he, too, must have the same symptoms and be suffering from PTSD. That sort of thing. Carelessness. Unthinking. Mind you, and I do have to admit this, my case was somewhat different insofar as – well, few people believe that a homosexual relationship can be anything more than a transient, flash-in-the-pan episode. They refuse to credit it with any intensity of emotion except on a very superficial level and hence, of course, it is well-nigh impossible for them to attribute anything as severe as trauma resulting from the breakdown, for whatever cause, of such a relationship. It is viewed, I'm sure, on a purely sexual level. Devoid of any natural emotion. Oh, yes, I did in fact. But even he, a good friend and a prominent psychologist, had trouble coming to terms with the fact that I was claiming to be traumatised by Peter's death. If it had been a Betty or a Gladys or a Petronella, for God's sake, he would have understood. No, he didn't *say* that. He didn't have to.

How? Ah, that was almost as traumatic. I remember the first thing I did was to remove every trace of Peter from the house. Every plate, every cup and mug he had used was smashed and thrown out. Every photograph destroyed. In a sort of frenzy. All in one morning. And it seemed to clear the air. I seemed to be doing something positive. Or so I convinced myself. I then had to get myself back into shape. I made out a list of menus of food I would force myself to eat, one for each evening. I made out a timetable, I have it somewhere if you want – No? Good. I doubt if I could put my hands on it. It's somewhere around – listing the things I would have to do. Such and such a time to shave, to bathe, to take a short walk, that sort of thing. I remember the very first step I took outside the door in, quite literally months, was when I sneaked out to have my hair cut. And I do mean 'sneaked'. I was truly petrified . . . No idea. None. None whatever. I suppose I imagined my mental condition might show on my face like warts and that people would stare at me. I think, too, that I feared everyone *knew* what had happened to me and that I might be viewed as some sort of freak. There's no doubt in my mind that overcoming that hurdle, actually *making* myself go out for something as mundane as a haircut, was tremendously significant in getting me back on a more or less even keel. From then on it was a case of simply making myself do all the normal things that had been natural to me, and to anyone else, before Peter's death. There are still things I cannot bring myself to do. Hah! As soon as I'd said that I knew you'd ask, and now, for the life of me I cannot think of anything. Things just crop up and I can recognise myself avoiding doing them. Certain music I can't listen to. Nothing that Peter liked. No. Just music that seems to evoke an image of him. Delius for some reason.

Yes. In a sense I do feel ostracised, but it's of my own doing, I'm sure. What I mean by that is – tell the truth, I'm not sure what I mean! Let me think. Well, I still have this feeling of guilt. I still find myself reduced to tears from time to time – less frequently now, thank God – for no apparent reason. Not great wailing, you understand. Just an incontrollable weeping. And sleeping is virtually an unknown quantity to me. Anyway, all that sets me apart, if you like, if only in my own way of thinking. You might say I ostracise myself. I feel, unreasonably, uncomfortable in company although I still struggle to overcome that. And I'm getting better at it even if I'm always relieved to get away and be by myself again no matter how enjoyable the company . . . Oh no. No, I've had no relationships of that nature since. Really could not. No, it's not from any sense of loyalty or of being faithful to Peter's memory. Nothing like that. I just don't *want* one. I don't want anyone getting too close to me, getting to know me too well. Ah, but this is quite different. I'm viewing this – I hope I'm not being impolite – viewing this as part of my – I nearly said rehabilitation – nothing like that – well, perhaps a bit like that – more of an exercise to see how far I was willing to go with a stranger. How much I would admit to . . . Quite well, I think, don't you? I've done better than I thought I would. Far better. I think we could allow ourselves a small drink, don't you? To celebrate whatever it is one celebrates in such cases.

No. I'll not practise again, I shouldn't think. That problem still has to be resolved. It's one I put on the long finger, however. I feel it would be obscene to go back to my practice and use my good ladies as sort of guinea-pigs to overcome *my* problems. What *will* I do? I don't honestly know. I don't tend to plan too far ahead, you see. Not any more. I used to be very meticulous about planning things, lists and lists, diaries filled with details of all my comings and goings. But not any more. I spend a couple of months each year in France now. A tiny village near Aix-en-Provence. I might start spending more time there. Maybe even sell up here and move there permanently. Oh no, nothing like that. I don't really believe in all that fresh start with a clean slate business. However, despite what many might say or think, the French do respect one's privacy. That's desperately important to me. Privacy. It always has been, but even more so now. The French don't try to jolly you along the whole time once you've made it clear you want to be left alone. That's something that has always shocked and appalled me – the way people, even people who you know to be kind, sensitive and understanding, can be so unashamedly intrusive when one is grieving. It's a frightful and unthinking impertinence, really. I'll always remember when my parents died – they died within two days of each other, incidently – the way people, even those who I would never have considered to be my friends, kept intruding, offering the most ludicrous snippets of advice. You know the sort of thing: God is good. He'll look after them. Time is a healer. All that twaddle. It really was the most insidious kind of harassment. At the time I couldn't have cared less about God's goodness or what particular miraculous powers time had to heal. That's why I like the French. They would never have presumed to behave like that. They respect sorrow as a very private emotion and allow the sorrower the room to grieve. The last thing I think the griever wants is to feel his grief is being taken away from him and placed in

90

the hands of some god in whom he might or might not believe.

Yes. Yes. I still grieve. Of course I do. It is a different pattern of grief. I don't tend to do it consciously any more. It has become a way of life. Part of my life. Like eating. Perhaps more like smiling. I do it when I think it's proper. Not all the time. Only when it's appropriate and even then without fully appreciating that I *am* doing it. Not until later. In a curious way I find it comforting, and I think I would feel bereft without it, but let's not get into that. That's another question altogether, I think.

Yes. I do think my being homosexual puts a different slant on the way I see things. Oh, I know it's fashionable to say we're *not* different – just the same as everyone else except in our sexual life. But I don't think that is true. We are different in the same way men and women are different. I don't mean physically, of course. Mentally. We *do* look at the world in a different way to heterosexual men. I think it's very natural that we should. For my own part I know I have a greater leaning towards the feminine emotions, and I thank God I do. It certainly has helped me. I feel, for example, no shame or embarrassment about crying. None whatever. And having been able to cry certainly enabled me to unleash an enormous amount of my pent-up sorrow. If I had been forced to restrain that with a totally male stiff upper-lip nonsense I don't know what would have happened. I might possibly have had a total breakdown. Women, too, have a certain stoicism which is an admirable quality. I think I have also. An acceptance of the divine will. The order of things. An acceptance that certain things must happen. An acceptance of fate, I suppose. Men don't, as a rule, in my experience, have that gift of acceptance. They seem determined, driven almost, to change. To impose their will . . . I really am getting away from the point. Tell you what. Let us have a glass of Madeira and drink to happier times ahead. For both of us. For all of us. I think that would be an appropriate toast, don't you? Happier times for all of us.

I have had two postcards from Arthur Dunlop, both from France. I do not know for certain but I think he has, as he said he might, moved there permanently. The second postcard read: 'Soldiering on. Regarded here as a most odd creature. Typical British eccentric and accorded the benign eye reserved for that well-nigh extinct species. With affection. Arthur.'

91

EIGHT

No energy, no interest, nothing

EOIN AND WINNIE McCOIST

The town of Lockerbie is only twelve miles from where I live. On the evening of Wednesday, 21 December 1988, Flight PA 103, a Pan Am Boeing 747 jumbo jet, registered number N739PA, disappeared from the radar screen at Prestwick air traffic control. The jumbo, with 259 passengers and crew aboard, was *en route* from London Heathrow to New York's John F. Kennedy airport. Without warning, the aircraft disintegrated at 31,000 feet. Until the flight's transponder return disappeared from the controller's radar screen, there had been no indication of any problem; the aircraft had been transferred as normal from London air traffic control (ATC) to Scottish and then on to Oceanic.

Primary radar tapes showed the aircraft breaking into five sections. There was no Mayday call, and those on the ground were unaware of the catastrophe six miles up for another three minutes, when parts of the plane, some now burning fiercely, ploughed into the town of Lockerbie, in Scotland. Wreckage and bodies were scattered over a wide area in six main locations. Most of the wreckage fell to the east of the A74 trunk road, and stretched over a six to eight-mile east-west path just over a mile wide. A severed wing tore a swathe of destruction through the south side of the town and a massive explosion made a crater 40 feet deep, 50 yards

93

long and 20 yards wide. Houses caught fire and four, in the direct path of the aircraft, simply disappeared in the explosion. The town's Sherwood Crescent was decimated with sixteen houses destroyed or rendered uninhabitable. The tail and rear fuselage plummetted on to the town's housing estate of Rosebank, catching the end of a terraced row of houses. The cockpit, remarkably intact, crashed three miles away at Tundergarth Hill. More than sixty bodies rained down on the local golf course, littering the fairways and bunkers. Other bodies landed in gardens, on rooftops, and even penetrated houses, ending up in attics and roof-spaces. The tail section landed twenty-one miles away near the Borders town of Langholm.

All those on board perished, and eleven local residents were killed, bringing the death toll to a total of 270. Debris from the aircraft was later discovered as far as eighty miles away, and the bodies of passengers were scattered over a ten-mile radius. The impact of such horror on the whole of Dumfries and Galloway, and particularly on the town of Lockerbie was, quite literally, unimaginable.

Of the twenty-eight women I contacted for possible inclusion in this book Winnie McCoist was one of only two who agreed to be interviewed, and then only on the stipulation that her husband be with her during all our conversations. Because of this I decided to transcribe the interview somewhat differently. I felt that Eoin McCoist's contributions were equally legitimate and interesting since he, clearly, was also a victim although officially he would be classed as a 'secondary' victim – someone suffering stress because of the traumatic stress experienced by another, usually a loved one. To me it seemed, in this case at least, that the line between primary and secondary was very fine. Eoin's responses are indicated by the use of italics.

Winnie McCoist is thirty-four, her husband three years older. They have two children, both of whom, fortunately, were staying with their grandparents on the night of the tragedy. The McCoist home is a bungalow within walking distance of the centre of Lockerbie town. They are very private people, wary of intrusion, and it took several months before they would agree to talk to me. They were the only ones to run a thorough check on me, contacting both my publisher and my agent. This, they explained, was because they were worried I might be from the press by whom they had already been 'badgered and brow-beaten', in particular in the days immediately following the disaster. Like many of the residents of the town, they had been dismayed and pained by what they described as the distortions that had been printed.

The interview was recorded in one sitting, lasting from two in the afternoon until just after seven o'clock in the evening. During all that time Winnie McCoist sat in approximately the same position, barely moving: very erect in an upright chair, her hands folded on her lap. Eoin McCoist sat beside her, more comfortably, in an armchair. He looked at her frequently, and from time to time would reach out and take one of her hands, squeezing it gently. When tea was offered it was he who went to the kitchen and made it; for most of his statements, he sought agreement from his wife.

You'll understand this is very difficult for us. Isn't it, Win?
     Yes.
     Even up to last night we were in two minds whether to go through with it or not. Why did we? Because – to set the record straight. It was Winnie's idea, wasn't it?
     Yes.
     We're all getting a bad name. Everyone in the town is. All that fighting about compensation as if that was going to help. Makes everyone sound greedy. We're not like that here. Sure, sure the money will help rebuild the homes that were destroyed but it won't rebuild the lives, will it?
     It's caused more trouble than anything else.
     Yes, it certainly has. Jealousy, too. Why should so-and-so get so much and someone else not get that amount.
     We feel the community's just being ripped apart.
     It is. It is. Yes, we were told to. Everyone was. But we never put in any claims for anything. What we want is to try and put the whole thing behind us and just get on with our lives as best we can. It's not easy that, you know, what with the enquiry going on and on, and all the haggling. Bad for the kids in particular.
     That's the worst thing. The children being hounded; although that's stopped mostly now. But it was terrible. And you know what children are like. They love the attention and all that. The press really used that. I'll never be able to forgive them for the way they behaved.

95

If we'd all been left alone we'd probably all be over it by now. It was that sort of place. People cared about each other. We could have managed. But it got to the stage when we couldn't even go to see a neighbour without being hounded by photographers.

And another thing: we felt we were being used like guinea-pigs or something. Everyone wanted to ask questions. They landed us with God alone knows what sort of people – you know, psychiatrists – that sort, all probing and not leaving us alone.

All we wanted was a little time to ourselves to grieve but they wouldn't give us that. Kept saying we should talk about it –

Get it out in the open, they said, didn't they?

We felt that we should show our respect for the dead by being quiet but, no, that wasn't the way they wanted it. Horrible.

And I think it's because of that, because we weren't allowed time to ourselves that there's so much difference in people. We've all changed, every last person in the town has changed. Some more than others. Some so you wouldn't really notice. But everyone's different in some way. And it'll never be like it was. That's why we're moving.

Yes. We decided to move up close to Eoin's parents.

Mostly for the kids. Let them have a normal life.

They never will here. Too many memories. Too much intrusion. Still. Even after all this time.

And something else. We just don't feel we fit in here any more. Winnie and me. Do we?

Not any more.

Why? Well, that's hard –

Me mostly –

No –

Yes, it is. Me mostly. Eoin's coping really well. But me, I don't seem to be able to be myself again. Always snapping at the children, or just sitting and saying nothing. Wanting to speak, mind, but finding nothing to say. I used to be interested in everything. But now I've no interest. No energy. Nothing. Like I'm not even alive half the time.

Oh, no. Not immediately. There was too much to do immediately after the accident. We had to help, didn't we? And we were all alright while we were helping. Doing something. It was later, maybe a week or so afterwards that it started to hit us.

It started with me not wanting to go out of the house, didn't it? I just couldn't get myself to go out any more. I had shopping to do but couldn't bring myself to go down to the shops.

More like you didn't want *to go to the shops, Win.*

Yes. Yes, that's right. Didn't seem any point. I mean, I knew there was a point – getting food in for Eoin and the children – but somehow I couldn't *see* the point of that – does that make sense?

You've got to understand that Winnie was really friendly with everyone. She loved going down the town for a chat and a gossip, didn't you? And then, not all at once, mind, slowly, gradually, she just stopped going out. There was one time she didn't go out for nearly six weeks. Not even into the garden. Never set foot outside the door, did you?

No. Just didn't want to. I kept telling myself I was being stupid, but it was as if I didn't believe myself. What did I do? Just sit here. Sometimes I'd sit here all day with the curtains drawn from the night before . . . No, I don't remember what I'd be thinking. Maybe I wasn't thinking at all. Maybe my mind was just blank. I don't know. And, then, the day would be gone and Eoin would be home and the children back from school and I'd still be sitting here wondering where the day had gone and what I'd done with it. Eoin had to do everything, didn't you? All the cooking and everything. I was useless.

You weren't yourself.

No, I wasn't.

And she had nightmares too. So even at night she didn't have any rest. That was half the trouble, I think. No rest night or day.

But you didn't either.

That was different. I had to keep going. *Had my job to do, hadn't I? That helped me a lot. It was* normal, *you see. Working. Getting away from things. Just working. Different for Winnie, just having nothing really to do.*

I had plenty to do if I'd wanted to do it.

Yes, but nothing that really had *to be done, if you know what I mean.*

Yes. Yes, I did go to the doctor. But – well, it was difficult. Everyone seemed to be going to the doctor. He was very busy. I think, too, that he didn't really know what was happening. Don't think I'm being critical. He was very kind and very understanding, but all this was new. Oh, what they call stress on a huge scale. And I didn't help him very

97

much. I couldn't. All I could do was say I had no energy and that I was sleeping badly. That wasn't much help to him, was it? Yes, he gave me some sleeping tablets and told me to give myself time.

Tablets helped her sleep but they didn't stop the nightmares.

That wasn't the doctor's fault.

I'm not saying it was. Just saying they didn't –

I know. I'm sorry, Eoin.

Anyway, things started getting worse for a while, didn't they? For a while, about three or four weeks, wasn't it, Winnie lost her memory completely. Couldn't remember the crash. Couldn't remember me or the kids. Couldn't remember any damn thing. She'd just sit and stare at nothing all day, and at night she wouldn't go to bed, just stay sitting in that chair where she'd been all day, staring at the wall or the curtains. We'd put the TV on but she didn't seem to watch that. But the thing was – later when she came to herself again – she said she hadn't lost her memory. You better explain that.

You want me to? Well, I could remember some things. I'll tell you what it was like exactly. An aunt of mine had a stroke and her mind went and all she could remember and talk about was her childhood. It was like as if she *was* a child again. Well, it was the same with me. I could distinctly remember everything about myself up to about the age of twenty, up to before Eoin and I were married anyway. It was like I *was* only twenty again. Nothing had happened after that. And the funny thing was, I was able to remember things from my childhood that I thought I'd really forgotten. Just silly little things of no importance. That's what it was like. I'd stopped living from the age of twenty. No, no, that's not it. I actually hadn't lived past twenty.

Yes. That's right. Just like that. One day her memory came back for no reason.

It was just like waking up from a dream.

That's actually what she said – I've been dreaming.

Yes, I did, didn't I?

Yes. We just carried on as if that blankness had never happened. Got to. What else was there for us to do?

No. There's been no relapses or anything.

And it seemed to help a bit too, didn't it? She was better for quite a while after that. Not completely better. But she didn't cry all the time. She used to

98

do that. Cry. And moan away to herself. But she stopped that. And started talking to us again, not just staring into space.

And the nightmares suddenly left me.

Yes.

I don't even have any dreams now, good or bad.

But you still can't sleep much.

No, but that doesn't matter. I get by on very little sleep. Yes, maybe that is why I've so little energy, but I think it's more than that. It's like – there's a word for it that escapes me – Yes. Apathy. It means no energy because you've lost interest, doesn't it? Something like that anyway. Interest? I don't honestly know.

Just nothing seems important to you now, does it, Win?

That's too simple. Of course things are important – the children, you, you're important, of course you all are. I can see and understand that certain things are important, very important, but I just can't seem to be that *interested* in them.

No, you ask what you want. Honestly. If we don't want to answer we'll say so. Tell you – I was going to say mind your own business, but we wouldn't say that. Just wouldn't answer. What was it you wanted to ask us? . . . Winnie's been asked that already. Haven't you, Win? One of those – what was she? – never did find out – one of those young lasses they sent around – some sort of student psychologist or something, I suppose. Didn't answer her. Why should we? None of her business at all. God knows what she'd have done with the information. Couldn't expose Win to that sort of questioning. Came with her clipboard and her questions all prepared. Some sort of survey, it was like. Like those soap-powder – you know, when they stop you on the street. Thought we'd be impressed with her being so matter-of-fact and business-like. But you could see she didn't really care. Not about us. About her survey she cared, but not about us, so we ran her off. There was a lot of that. People running round collecting data – that's the word they used – data – but not caring what we were going through. Anyway, to answer your question: no, we don't any more. We had been planning one more kid, but we've given up on that idea for the time being at least.

I can't help remembering there were children on that plane – children – children.

All right, Win. All right. Let me go and make us all a cup of tea.

99

What no one seems to understand is that we've had no real chance to get over it all. It was such a big tragedy, I mean. Aroused so much interest. And then the politics of it all started to come into play with the enquiry. Those of us who were really affected by the whole episode – you know, the relatives of those who were killed and all of us here in the town – were overlooked, had to take a back seat if you like, while the lawyers and the politicians started their haggling.

The way I see it is that it doesn't matter *who* did it, *who* was responsible. It was done and that's an end to it. Tell me, what's more important – that some terrorists are made to appear in court and be found guilty in the eyes of the world or that we, the people here in the town, are allowed to pick up the pieces and get our lives back into some sort of shape once again? It doesn't matter to us if they were Libyan or Iraqi or Iranian. What difference does that make? Or where they're tried? Or even if they're tried. How will that help anyone? How will that stop people grieving?

Doesn't seem to be any point in it, does there? Just dragging it on the way they do, keep reminding people of it instead of letting it ebb away. Look, don't take this the wrong way, will you, but I don't think the number of people killed matters. I mean, to any family, one death is terrible, and when that happens you don't keep going over and over it, putting yourself through the pain of that death for ever. You grieve in private. You cry, don't you, but to yourself. And you give yourself the time to get over it, let the hurt fade and re-member the good things about that person. Well, that hasn't been allowed to happen here. And even when we are coming to terms with it – what happens? It'll be the anniversary, or something – like that solicitor getting killed in the car accident the way he was – and it's all front-page news again.

Like we told you, that's why we *have* to move away. That's why *we* have to move away. What other people do is up to them.

Yes. Some people here are able to cope with it all. Or they say they can. They go about the day as if they can, anyway. But I'm sure – absolutely sure – that you'd find a load of people who were suffering just like Win and me if they'd only admit it. But it's hard to admit something like this. Makes you look weak, doesn't it? Nobody wants to be made to look weak. And if we feel the way we do – what about the people who woke up to find bodies in their gardens? What must they be going through? But who asks them? Who goes and tries to help them?

It'll never be like it was.

Can't be.

And we can't be.

No.

No, we can't know that – can't really know if moving is going to help. All we can do is hope that things will be better. It's *got* to be, doesn't it?

You know the stupid thing? I might be wrong about this, but it's like as if we were being made to feel guilty for what happened. I can't explain it, but it's doing nothing but damage. Like, somehow, everyone in the town dragged that plane down on top of us. And some of us got killed and some of us survived, and the survivors are being made to feel guilty for the ones who died. Does that make any sense? Probably not. It's just a feeling. Nothing else. But we've got to live with it. And it doesn't make it any easier the way everyone's being bullied and pushed into cashing in on it. Claim this. Claim that. They kept coming round here telling us what we should do, telling us what we should demand, telling us that we should make someone pay. How could a man use any of that money? Wouldn't that really be blood money? What would you buy with it? Christ Almighty, no matter what you bought you'd have to think – I don't know – I'm driving this nice new car, or looking at that nice new television, or wearing these fancy new clothes because of someone else's death. But you couldn't live like that, could you? And respect yourself at the same time. We couldn't anyway. Like grave-robbing. That's what I think it's like. Plundering graves and that's all wrong.

It's made everyone different.

Yes. That's right. Everyone. I guarantee you there's not a single soul in the town who's the same as they were before. No, you're right. You couldn't expect them to be. Not the way things were handled. All the interference. All those know-alls telling us what was best for us – as if they could know what was best for us. You know. if we'd just been left alone, left to ourselves without all that interference we'd have had a better chance of getting back to the way we were. Tell you something – when I saw the faces of those American parents on the telly – when they'd been told compensation would be paid, you know – I felt sick. Turned my stomach. They were so pleased. The money made them pleased. They'd lost people they loved and they were pleased to be getting money for that. I don't know. I don't know what way

101

people think any more. That's all I'm saying. Can't fathom people out at all. And Win's the one who's supposed to be sick. Crazy, isn't it?

All right, Eoin.

Yes. Sorry. Just makes me so angry . . . Pardon? Oh. Well, I don't know. Don't really expect any more, do we, Win? We don't expect Win to get completely better. We hope. That's it. We hope. We don't expect it. And she is getting better, aren't you, pet?

Yes. I am. Very slowly though. Very slowly.

Okay. Slowly. But that's better than not at all, isn't it. We'll be all right in the end. I know we will. We'll muddle through by ourselves, like they say. Muddle through and come out the other end. What else is there to do, tell me?

No, Eoin. You stay there. I'll see Mr Power to the door. I'd like to do that. Yes. I'm sure.

The McCoist family have now moved close to Eoin's parents' home in Ayrshire. They have both my telephone number and address but, as yet, have not contacted me again.

NINE

Just dirty, that's how I feel, dirty

PAULINE CHESTERTON

Pauline Chesterton is twenty-nine, blonde-haired, slim, and quietly spoken. She lives alone in a two-roomed basement flat near the centre of York. The curtains in the room facing the street are always drawn; the light burns there twenty-four hours a day.

In 1984 Pauline Chesterton lived in London. On the night of 17 July a man broke into her flat and viciously raped her several times. He held a knife to her throat and, having raped her, used the knife to inflict a long, jagged wound the length of her left cheek, saying it was his calling card. A month after the attack Pauline left her job with a bank and moved to York. She is at a loss to explain why she chose York: she had never been there before. She thinks perhaps that is, in fact, one of the reasons. She now works part-time, mornings only. Afternoons and evenings are usually spent alone in her flat, although recently she has started going to matinees at the cinema with a friend from work. She is a voracious reader, and it was after reading one of my books that she decided to contact me through the publisher. 'To this day I don't know why. Something about the way you wrote, things you said, the way you put things made me feel I could talk to you, and I've wanted to talk to someone for years.' In fact, what Pauline had actually wanted was someone to *write* to. At the time neither she nor I had any idea that I would be doing this particular book: it was only when this book was conceived that we arranged to meet.

I never did tell you about the curtains, did I? It seems such a silly thing to tell anyone. Makes me sound very silly, not letting the light in. I chose the basement flat because of the bars on the windows, and the curtains – well, that's obviously so that no one can see in. Even if they got through the bars they wouldn't know who was on the inside, would they? It might be a karate expert with a couple of Rottweilers. That's part of it. The other part is this – this scar – it's much less obvious than it was but, just the same, keeping the place darkish makes it even harder to see. For me to see anyway. No, I know it's not obvious the way I do my hair, but I *know* it's there. I used to keep running my fingers down it. I don't do *that* any more, which is something. Just learning to live with it, I suppose.

Yes. Yes, I did try talking to someone else, but that was a long, long time ago. Someone I thought I knew very well. Someone I thought would understand. But, you know, it's very strange how people react to something like this. Rape. It makes *them* so uncomfortable. Like as if I was trying to rape them in a way. Trying to draw them into my anger, anyway. And they don't want that. Nobody does. Yes, I know that there's a crisis line and all that sort of thing now, but – I don't know – I didn't want that. I didn't want pity, I suppose, and that's what I believed they'd give me. Pity. Something you give to a dog that's been injured on the street. Didn't want that at all. No, I've no idea what I wanted. That was the trouble. I wanted to curl up and just disappear, I think. Wanted most of all to wake up and find it had been a nightmare. But I always had this to remind me. No matter how hard I tried to hide it with make-up, it was always there to remind me. Police? Good heavens, no! Yes, I *thought* about it, of course, but never as a serious option. Why? Because – fear, I imagine. Not of them but of what I might have to go through. I mean, the whole point in going to the police would have been to get him caught but that would have meant a court case and publicity and everything like that. To be truthful: in a ridiculous way I didn't want him caught, you see. By not catching him I could hope that the whole thing would go away. Anyway, whatever the reason, I didn't ever seriously think about going to the police. Especially not after my friend couldn't understand. That was awful. A great shock. After that I was really on my own. That was when I decided to leave London. I know it was running away, but that's what one does when one is frightened, isn't it? Run away. Run as fast and as far as you can.

No, I honestly don't mind talking about it now. Like I told you in my letters, I can be quite clinical about it, in fact. I know . . . you said that . . . but I suppose I found that particular bit a little funny – not funny funny – sort of weird funny – to try and make myself accept it all. I only thought about it when that friend asked if it hurt, meaning physically. My friend knew I was a virgin at the time and must have thought that would have made it hurt. But it didn't. He had the most ridiculous little thing. Maybe that's why he had to rape rather than – you know. Maybe he was ashamed of it. Anyway, from time to time I think about how tiny it was and that just seems funny – weird funny as I said. The rest wasn't funny at all, though. It was so – so unexpected. You read about this sort of thing happening, and you think how awful, but you never really associate it with anything that will happen to you. And then it does. Out of the blue. And from then on you keep going over and over it in your mind, and you keep remembering things, little things, irrelevant things, like – Well, I was brought up Catholic and one of the things I kept thinking was I'm not doing this, I'm not doing this, as if I was trying to convince God that I was not agreeing to the rape, as if He didn't know. Pardon? Oh. Yes. No, I don't mind. You know most of it already from my letters anyway.

Well, I came home from work. I shared the flat in Clapham but my flatmate was on holiday so I had the place to myself. She was coming home the next day so I had decided to spend the evening tidying everything up. I remember it was very hot. I decided to take a shower and stripped down to my underwear, then I changed my mind and decided to do the housework first and then have a shower. I remember I opened the window wide – a big window looking out on to the street. He told me that he'd seen me open the window. Said he'd watched me open the window. Anyway, I got everything done, and had my shower. I fixed myself something to eat: salad, I think, and then settled down to watch TV. I can't remember now what it was but there was something on that evening that I particularly wanted to see. I remember that clearly because some of the girls from the bank wanted me to go out with them that evening and had made a great deal out of my wanting to watch this programme. It must have been some soap or something. Maybe not. Maybe just some one-off thing that I wanted to see. Then I went to bed.

You'd think you'd forget things after all this time, wouldn't you? I don't mean forget all about it, of course not that. But you'd think the details would fade somewhat. They don't, you know. They really don't. If anything they become clearer. No, that's not true either. They separate themselves. That's it. They're no longer fuzzy. They stand out by themselves. Very frightening, that can be. Used to be. No, I don't believe so. I really don't believe it *frightens* me to think about it now. It angers me. Yes, makes me really angry. Oh, don't get me wrong. I'm still terrified that I might be raped again. That never goes away, I don't think. But the little details aren't frightening. I can't explain it any better than that. Let me think a minute. Well, for my twenty-first birthday my mother and Dad gave me a little chiming carriage clock. You know the ones. Not an antique. A modern imitation. I kept it on my dressing-table. It chimed only the hour, not the quarters. I can remember that when he . . . he'd been mauling me for about, I don't know exactly, about ten minutes I suppose, when the clock chimed two. For ages after that everytime the clock chimed two I'd get this panic feeling. Real panic. Start shaking and go all weepy. I had to stop the chime in the end. Had to. Found myself actually waiting for it. Waiting to panic. There was nothing I could do about it. That was the worst thing. Nothing I could do. I'd be in bed, not sleeping, just waiting for those chimes.

Oh, through the window. Very easily, it seems. The flat below had a small bay window and the roof of that jutted out about a foot. He just climbed on to that and in the window. He even thanked me for leaving the window open. Made it sound like I'd issued an invitation. 'Thank you for leaving the window open,' he said. He said that when he first woke me up and again when he was leaving. Twice. Not with any menace or anything. Very polite. No, I never heard a thing. And he'd been in the flat for quite a while before he attacked me. Been through some of my drawers. No, he didn't take anything. I don't know what he was doing. Just looking at my things, I suppose.

That's the strangest, most frightening thing, I think. I've no idea whatever what he looked like. That made it worse later because any man that looked at me made me wonder if it was him. Any man. And that was stupid since I did know certain things. Like, for example, he was white and youngish and quite small. But even if a black man looked at me, I'd wonder. If an old man looked at me, I'd wonder. If a huge, tall man looked at me, I'd wonder. But that's all I really knew: white, young, smallish. And his hair was short and he had hard hands. Oh, and he smelled clean. Crazy, I remember thinking, 'At least he's clean', as if that really mattered. There's so many things that race through your mind. It's almost as if – well, as if the actual rape isn't that bad when you can start thinking 'please don't let him mark me or kill me'. Or maybe it's to get your mind off what he's doing that you start thinking of other things. About him being clean and all. Another thing I found. I found myself listening – I mean *really* listening – to every word he said, but because of everything that's happening you can't quite make out what he's saying, so what he *is* saying gets much more important. I don't know. I can't explain it.

Oh, yes. Oh, yes. I remember *exactly* what his first words were. I didn't wake up until he was on top of me and he said, 'Don't scream. Don't do anything stupid. I don't want to kill you but I can. This is a knife.' Then he prodded my neck with his knife. Just a small prick to prove he had one. I must have done something, I don't know, relaxed or something, because then he said, 'That's good. That's better. Thank you for leaving the window open.'

Struggle? No. No, I don't remember that I did struggle. I'm sure I didn't. I think I was just too frightened to struggle, to put up any sort of fight. I didn't want to get killed. I kept thinking, let him do it and then he'll go away. That's all you can think about. Surviving. I do remember thinking, at least I *think* I thought, he's going to rape you but you'll get over that, just don't do anything to make him angry and hurt you. I say I *think* I remember thinking that because I can't honestly be sure whether I was actually thinking that at the time or whether it was something I told myself I'd been thinking later. You know how it is. You know you're somewhere and someone makes a smart remark and it's only ages afterwards, when it's too late, you think of an answer you should have given back. Like that. I know that some of the things that came into my mind afterwards were things I *should* have done and said, but if I did say or do them I can't honestly be sure.

Anyway – anyway he raped me for the first time. It was very quick. Really quick. And – look, I'm going to tell you something that you could take the wrong way – you know what I actually thought? I thought something like, 'Is that all? What are you making such a fuss about?' Isn't that terrible? I suppose it was the relief that he hadn't done anything – well, weird, I suppose. You read all about those things that men do. I suppose I'd all sorts of things going through my mind, things he *might* do, that when he didn't do them I was just relieved. And I found myself agreeing with him. God, when I think about it! You see, when he was finished he lay on top of me still and kept saying wasn't that great, tell me it was great, tell me you loved it, tell me it was terrific, stuff like that, and I could hear myself saying, yes, it was great, yes, it was terrific. He said, 'I'm really good, aren't I?' and I said, 'Yes, you're really good'. Mad. Mad. Mad. Made everything all the worse, of course. Maybe he knew that. I don't know. Like, by agreeing with him it made it seem like I was – what's the word – condoning what he was doing. Complying. But, then anyway, I didn't care what I did so long as I could get him to leave. I kept thinking he's done it now and he'll go. It's over. He'll go now.

No, he didn't. He just stayed there on top of me. Very still. Not moving at all. Not saying anything. I thought he'd fallen asleep, really. But he hadn't. I must have moved because immediately he stuck the knife into my neck again and said something like – I don't know exactly – don't move or stay still or something. You know what was awful? I could hear things, normal things, going on outside. Like cars passing. Doors being closed. Even some music playing somewhere. It was like as if nobody cared what was happening to me. I felt no one should be doing anything except trying to save me. If they didn't know what was happening – and they didn't obviously – they *should* have known. It was their business to know. It was like when my dad died. He died at home from a stroke. Well, he was lying dead and outside life went on. I felt life shouldn't be going on. *Everyone* should have been mourning, but they weren't, of course. Well, it was the same –

108

something the same, anyway – as that. It was the feeling of – well, isolation, I suppose, of being so alone and vulnerable and incapable – that's it, incapable – that was so awful.

Three times. Three times. He tried four but couldn't. It was getting light by then anyway. Just a little. I think that's what made him angry. That he couldn't do it again, either because he *couldn't* or he was afraid it might get so light I'd see what he looked like. I don't know which. But all the time he kept wanting to be told how great it was and how good he was at it. That seemed more important to him than anything else. You know, I've thought about that a lot. And I think that the actual sex didn't mean that much to him: it was me telling him how good he was that mattered. Anyway, like I said, he got angry when he couldn't do it any more for whatever reason. Not wild angry. Not ranting. Just cold angry. Vicious, I suppose. That was when he did this. Cut me. I didn't even know he'd cut me until after he'd gone and I saw all the blood. He just ran the knife down my cheek and said, 'That's my calling card', and then, really quickly, he was gone. The window? No, out the door. He walked, ran, out the door.

Yes, certainly, that was the first thing that came to mind. To scream. But just as quickly I thought that if I screamed people would find out what had happened to me and I didn't want that. I don't really. I suppose I thought they'd – that they wouldn't believe me – that I'd asked for it – I don't know. I just know that I didn't want anyone to find out. So, in a way, I became very practical about it. I actually sat on the edge of the bed and worked things out. Worked out what I should do. Have a shower. That was the first thing. Then, I remember, change the sheets on the bed. Close the window. I was thinking those things when I noticed the blood dripping from my face. I went into the bathroom and just stood looking at myself. For ages. Not doing anything. Not trying to stop the blood or anything. Just looking. You know, that scar, well, the cut as it was then, was worse, far worse, I think, than the rape. That's how it struck me at the time. I suppose I was lucky that he hadn't made a deep cut. Just broken the skin really. Enough to leave this scar but it wasn't deep. Nothing that needed stitches. I don't think I could have coped with that – having to explain how and everything.

109

How I got it. Not like a bruise you could pass off as having fallen down or bumped into a door. Anyway, I didn't want *anyone* to see me. And it wasn't just because of my face. I felt that everything that had happened would show somehow. That people would be able to *see* I'd been raped. I know that wasn't sensible, but that's the way it was. Just because I knew I expected everyone else to know. No, I don't think so. I don't think shame came into it then. It did later, but not then. I don't think I was even angry. Not really angry. I just felt dirty. Really filthy. That how I still feel, when I think about it. Dirty. I know I spent over an hour in the shower just scrubbing myself. I used my fingers trying to *peel* the dirt off. Like I could take it off in strips. Awful.

Well, I had to. Had to make some sort of explanation for my face. She was my flatmate so I couldn't avoid her. I avoided work, saying I had the flu or something. Yes, flu I think. So I told her I'd been out and a fight had started and me and a few other people got cut. I know she didn't believe me. She knew I wouldn't have been likely to go anywhere where there would have been *that* sort of fight. But I kept insisting it was true so she let it go. She couldn't do anything else. Oh, no. I'd managed to patch it up myself. I used TCP first. Then some Germoline and plasters. Nothing, and I mean nothing would have persuaded me to go near a hospital.

I stayed off work for a week. That was my intention anyway. But then came the day when I was supposed to go back, and I found that I simply couldn't, and that was when the real trouble started. For me. It was the first time, you see, when I'd have to start getting back to normality. Up to that I just stayed indoors. Now I'd have to go out. And I simply couldn't. And when I realised that I couldn't I started having a load of other problems. I started feeling his hard hands crawling all over me again. Night and day. I practically lived in the shower trying to get the feel of him off me. And I kept crying all the time. Even when I wasn't really thinking about anything. I'd just find myself crying. You know how they talk about tears of joy and tears of anger and all that? Not with me. It was just tears. Tears all the time.

So, I made another excuse to the bank to put them off for a while. They were very good about it. I kept saying I'd be back in a few days even though I knew full well that I wouldn't. I knew I'd *never* go back.

Yes, I think it was. It must have been, mustn't it? It must have been then that I decided to move away from London, but I don't even remember really thinking about it. It was a bit like I just packed my clothes and went rather than working it out. I must have thought it out though, because I left my flatmate my bits of furniture and things. The clock. My blankets. Just packed my clothes and went.

York? I've no idea. Just fixed on it. Never been here before. Knew nothing whatever about it except that there was a chocolate factory here. That too was a bit like I just arrived here without giving it any thought. I supposed I imagined that the people here were less likely to *see* I'd been raped. Mad, isn't it? But that's how it was. I was lucky I had a little money that Dad had left me. Not much but enough to get by on for a while. So I got this flat and I've been here since. My prison, really. No, that's not fair. Maybe I've made it a bit of a prison but that's not the flat's fault.

For ages, at first, I lived on practically nothing, trying to make the money last. It would have been better, really – I can say this with hindsight – if I'd have had no money. Then I would have been forced to get out and about if only to keep myself alive. But as long as I could pay the rent and get enough food to live on I couldn't even start to get back to any sort of normality. Those shopping expeditions! For food. God, they were horrendous. I used to dive into the shop, throw the first things that came to hand into the basket, dash up and pay for them, and race home, back here, again. I can tell you I ate some strange things during that time, but it just didn't seem to matter. Then I was down to my last few pounds and I had to do something, so I managed to get this job as a waitress part-time in a café. Just mornings, so it's easy. Coffee. Sandwiches. Things like that. I must be quite good at it because they keep asking me to work full-time. Maybe I will, one day. I'm getting a little more confident. Even went to the cinema with one of the other waitresses the other afternoon. But usually I'm by myself.

Like it? Being alone all the time? Yes. Yes, I do. That's not true. I hate it. I like it and hate it. What I mean is, I'd like to have people, friends, about me but I know I couldn't stand that, that's why I hate it. I like it because, well – because – I don't really know. Just being by myself means – means – I don't have to be afraid of anyone finding out, I suppose. Oh, yes. I'm still terrified that someone might find out. I

111

know that's unreasonable. I *know* it is, but that doesn't make any difference. Don't worry, I've thought about this over and over and over. I can tell you one conclusion I've come to. It's a crazy one. Quite mad. Well, it's this: you know he thanked me for leaving the window open? Well, I keep remembering that, and I keep wondering if, maybe, I did leave the window open on purpose. Now, I *know* I didn't. Of course I didn't. But I keep hearing him thanking me and the truth of the matter is, I keep wondering that if in some way I might be responsible for all that happened . . . I told you it was crazy. I don't just mean responsible. I mean guilty for what happened. You know, even now, every night when I go to bed I think about that night. I can hear every word he said, every sound he made, his breathing and grunting, and worst of all I can hear myself telling him how good he was. And on really bad nights I can actually *hear* my own voice saying the words, and sometimes they sound so convincing I wonder if I meant them. If, in some horrible way, I enjoyed it . . . I'm sorry. No, I'll be all right. Really, I will. I told you I get like this sometimes. I'll be all right in a minute.

Sorry about that. It's just I never said all that before. Thought about it yes, but never actually said it out loud. Came as a bit of a shock. Yes, I *do* know that. I *know* it's just some sort of reaction and a bit of my imagination playing up, but it doesn't really matter what the cause of it is. I still think it and have to live with it. That's the wicked thing he did. Making me live with it all. Sometimes I really do think it would have been better if he had killed me. Kinder. Kill me outright and not just leave me to die this way. Or just kill part of me. I don't know what I mean, really. I'm not really living, am I? Existing more like. That's it. I exist from day to day but I don't live from day to day like I should. There's a difference. I think so. Don't enjoy being alive at all. Not that I *want* to be dead, but I might as well be. That's what I think sometimes when I get very depressed.

No. No. I know I'll never get married. Just couldn't. Couldn't stand it. That's another thing I hate him for. I always dreamed of having children of my own. Even had some names picked out. Ruth and Sarah. David and Paul. Those were my favourites. Somehow I always thought I'd have four children – two boys and two girls. Just a fantasy,

I know, but it's the way I used to think of it. But now . . . For months
– far longer than was necessary – I remained petrified that he might
have made me pregnant. I really don't know what I'd have done then.
An abortion, I suppose, but that's awful. But I couldn't have had the
baby, could I? I might have ended up hating that too, and that would
have been unforgivable. But he didn't make me pregnant. Small mercy,
I suppose. But no, I'll never get married. Never go with a man again.
That's how I feel now at any rate. I couldn't. Just could not.

Thank you. Yes. I know I'm quite nice-looking. Even with the scar
because I can cover that with the way I do my hair. The men who come
into the café have made passes at me, the way men do, so I know I'm
reasonably presentable. I hated it at first when they tried to chat me up.
Made me feel sick. Made me shake all over. I just ignore it now. Trained
myself not to hear it. Where was I? – oh, yes. I was saying – it's not that
I think – you know – that any man I went out with might recoil or
whatever when he saw my face. It's – well, if you really want to know,
it's the dirtiness I feel. It's honestly like a disease of some sort. Like I'm
afflicted with a disease of some sort. Something awful. Something
transmissible. Like AIDS in a way. I think I might pass it on. Pass what
on? Well, the dirt or the sickness or whatever it is. All right. All right.
I *know* it's madness and that I'm being – over-sensitive or something.
But it's the way I am. The way I believe I'll always be. So I keep myself
to myself and don't have to make explanations to anyone. Don't have
to reject anyone or worry that I might be rejected. I just don't want to
cause anyone any harm. Myself? Yes. You could look at it that way –
that I'm harming myself, but that doesn't really matter any more. Not
to me. I can live with me as I am. Try to anyway. No, I do. I do manage
to live with myself. What's left of me. Actually, that's just the point. I'm
not really living with myself. I'm living with this new person, this
person I've become, this stranger. Takes some getting used to, but you
can get used to anything in time. That's what they tell me anyway. Well,
I'm beginning to get used to this stranger, getting to know her. Can't
say I like her a lot, but we all have our faults. Is this all gibberish? You
wouldn't tell me if it was anyway, would you? No, you wouldn't. Would
you really? All right. I believe you. I find myself doing that sometimes
– sitting here and talking away to myself, arguing with myself, out
loud. I'm not really talking to *myself* though. I'm chatting to the

stranger, to the new me. Oddly enough, it helps. Gets everything out into the open. That would be really nice. To really get everything out into the open. Anyway, the important point is that I know what I'm doing now. I know I'm just using this other me, so to speak, as a way of talking things out. And that's an improvement in itself, I think. You mightn't think so, but I do. You might be saying to yourself that I really am quite, quite mad. But I honestly don't think I am. I'm just doing what I have to do to cope. Simple as that. Learning to cope in my own little way, and you can't expect much more of me than that, can you?

Three months after the interview I was again in York and called to see Pauline to find out how she was getting on. It was a mistake. I should not have done so. She would not open the door to me, and asked me to go away. She told me that she had said all she wanted to say and wanted, now, to be left alone. It was only then that I fully realised what an enormous amount of courage it had taken for her to speak to me at all. For that I thank her, and apologise for what must have seemed like an unwarranted intrusion.

TEN

Football's shit now

BRENDAN KEYES

The Hillsborough tragedy has been well documented. On 15 April 1989 the two teams, Liverpool and Nottingham Forest, met in the FA Cup semi-final in Sheffield Wednesday's stadium at Hillsborough.

The crowd, as expected, was enormous, but who was responsible for the horrific event that followed is still unclear. There have been accusations and counter-accusations, but the most likely reason for the accident seems to be that the gates allowing access to the centre section of the West Stand were not closed once that section was filled. Fans anxious to see the kick-off continued to swarm in, setting off a chain reaction, causing those at the front of the West Stand to be crushed since they could not escape on to the pitch because of the crowd barriers.

The recent death of Tony Bland, who had been in a coma since the accident, brought the total of those killed to ninety-five. One hundred and seventy others were physically injured. How many still suffer traumatic stress from the incident remains to be assessed.

Brendan Keyes lives in Bootle with his parents. He is an only son. He is in his early twenties, but has the haunted, haggard look of a man far older than that.

On 15 April he travelled to Hillsborough with two friends who were also avid Liverpool supporters. They were shepherded into the West Stand, but became separated in the crowd.

My meeting Brendan came about by accident. I was in Liverpool researching child abuse and homelessness for a novel I was writing. Tony Speed, one of the young men I interviewed for that book, had also been at Hillsborough, and made some remark about being lucky it hadn't had that much effect on him. When I asked him what he meant, he told me about a friend of a friend of his who was still suffering from the effects of the disaster, someone who was 'shattered', as he put it. He was talking about Brendan.

When the time came to write this book I managed to contact Tony Speed again, and it was through him that Brendan and I met. Without his help I do not think Brendan would have spoken to me. It was, I believe, only after Tony had assured him that I wasn't 'mucking about', and told him that he, Tony, had spoken to me about his situation and had not found the experience too harrowing, that Brendan finally, after some months, agreed to talk to me.

The first thing I'll tell you – you got that thing running? – okay, well, the first thing I'll tell you is that football's shit now. For me, anyway. Just plain shit. Usen't to be, though. Used to be the greatest thing in the whole world. All I lived for, my mam used to say. And my dad. If only you'd put as much energy into your work as you do into that football you'd be a millionaire in no time. That's what Mam always said. That's when I was working, of course. And Dad agreed with her like he always does. Great one for keeping the peace my dad is. Agrees with anything as long as it keeps the peace. In the house, I mean. Outside he's different. Pretty aggressive he is outside. But he always agrees with Mam so she thinks she's getting her own way. I've picked up on that, too. Makes life easier. So I agree with her all the time. Like, see all those marks on the wall and the way the paper's torn? That's where I had all my posters. Hundreds of them. Well, dozens anyway. Lots of them signed. All Liverpool, of course. Best team in the world. Used to be. Best supporters, anyway. Still. And souvenirs. Loads of them, I had. Pride and joy, they were. Pride and joy. Just ripped them off any old how. That's why the paper's all torn. But what I was going to tell you was Mam often says, 'You've got to do something about that room of yours, Brendan, it's a disgrace', and Dad'll agree and say, 'Yes, why don't you go get some paper and redecorate it?', and I'll say, 'Sure, yes, must do that', and then I'll forget about it – no, not forget, just not do anything about it, and *Mam* will forget about it till the next time it comes into her head, maybe months later, and then we'll just go through all that crap again. That's how it goes. Same with everything, if you want to know. Just putting everything off till tomorrow and making sure tomorrow doesn't come. Anyway, you should have seen the stuff I had. Cost me an arm and a leg. Used to swap things with my mates, too. Like I'd find two of something somewhere and, for sure, only want one, so I'd do a deal with the other one for something I didn't have. Like they do with stamps, you know? Even managed to get a ball they used in training. Practically slept with that thing. And had one of Kenny's tops. Well, I was told it was one of his. Got if off Daffy – Tommy Eider, get it? – so I couldn't swear it *was* really one of Kenny's. Can't believe much of what Daffy says. Tell you anything, he would. Sell you anything, too. His mother if he could get someone stupid enough to pay for her. Just having you on. She's okay, really. Let's think what else. Photos. Hundreds of them and I do mean hundreds. Some I took or my mates took. Some put out by the club. Hundreds. Now? Nothing. Not one effing thing. Burned the lot, didn't I? Seemed the right thing to do. Been indecent to sell them. Yeah, could have given them away. But that didn't seem right either. Not at the time, anyway. Couldn't be sure they'd be appreciated right, and sure as hell couldn't go and make money out of them. That'd be sick. Really sick. Like burning them was proper. Respectful. Like they do with bodies in some countries, don't they? India and places. That's what I've heard anyway. Mates said I was crazy. Couldn't understand me at all. Doesn't matter, though. Certainly not now. Don't see them any more, do I? Can't be bothered. Tell you the truth, I don't understand how they can still go to the matches. Like watching the boys playing in a graveyard. That's how I see it. Wrong. All wrong. No, I never go. Haven't since it happened. How could I? And don't even watch it on telly. Don't want to know the results. Don't want to know anything about it. Nothing. Just doesn't happen any more as far as I'm concerned. Funny. Used to really look forward to Saturdays. Get all steamed up. Big day of the week, it was. Now – shit, I hate it. Don't come out of my room at all

117

on Saturdays. Lock myself in. Heard Mam say I was trying to keep the ghosts out. Maybe she's right. Don't think of it like that myself though. Ghosties, she called them. She does that. Doggies. Catties. Horsies. Ghosties. It's the way she talks. Dunno why. Just her way. Anyway, come to think of it now, right now I mean, she's wrong. Can't keep her ghosties out by locking the door. Stupid. They're in here already. All the time. And in here – in my head. No, doesn't worry me. They're okay. Don't cause me no bother. Get used to them, don't you? Get used to anything if you put your mind to it. You know that book that starts, 'It was the best of times, it was the worst of times'? That surprised you, didn't it, eh? Yeah, well, don't make too much of it. Haven't read it. Just heard it on some quiz show. Keeps coming up, that one does. Dickens, wasn't it? *Tale of Two Cities*. Yes. Anyway, sort of applies to me in a way. They really were the best of times as far as I was concerned. Then that fuck-up happened and it all became the worst of times. Make sense? Good. Does to me. Maybe I'm not explaining it right, but you know what I mean. Well, *I* know what I mean and I think that's what matters. Not being cheeky or anything. Don't take it that way, will you? Good. That's okay then.

No, I don't mind. Honest. Been through it loads of times. Tell the truth it's better with you. Why? Let's think. Well, like when I went to that psychiatrist – my mam fixed that up through the doc, thought I needed it, both of them. Well, Mam did and the doc agreed. Like I told you, Mam always gets her own way sometimes – well, when I was telling that psychiatrist everything it was like he was waiting to jump on me. Waiting, he was, for something *significant*. That was the word he liked. Oh, *that's* significant, don't you think, he'd say. Like he was just waiting for my significant sayings all the time. Scared the shit out of me. You, though, you're just hoping I say something. That's different, isn't it? Sure, I guess you'd be disappointed if I didn't tell you what you want to hear but – what am I trying to say? – yes, well, you don't *have* to have anything significant. You can switch that little thing off and toddle away with no skin off your nose. But that psychiatrist. He *had* to have something. Couldn't do his job without it, I suppose. Feel he'd failed or something. So, don't mind having a natter with you. You use it, you use it. You don't, you don't. No harm done. Nobody hurt. No big deal.

No pressure. Make no difference, no real difference, one way or the other, right? Sessions? Jeez, dunno. Can't remember. Lost count. Four. Maybe five. Maybe even six. Lost count. Didn't really care, you see. Just went along with it to keep the peace. Yeah, he told me I had this thing PTSD. Hang on, don't know if he did tell me. Maybe he told Mam and she told me. Dunno. Someone told me, that's all I know. Me? Just said something like 'great' or maybe 'terrific', you know, something a bit cheeky. Didn't know what they were talking about, did I? There was nothing wrong with me as far as I was concerned. Their problem, not mine. Remember Mam saying I wasn't to worry. Couldn't understand that. I *wasn't* worrying. They were doing all the worrying as far as I could see. She said everything would be all right. Stupid that was. Everything *was* all right. Started getting up my nose after a bit, it did. All that fussing about nothing. All I wanted was to be left alone. All I want still, really. Sorry. Don't mean you. Just generally. Just let everyone piss off and leave me be. Not too much to ask is it? Don't cause no trouble, I don't. Don't mean to, anyway.

You want a cup of coffee or something? Tea? No? Okay. No, I'm okay. Just had some soup stuff before you came. Marmite, I think. Just thought you might – okay then.

Well, four of us went. The same four of us that always went to matches together unless something serious cropped up like a world war or an atomic explosion or something. There was me and Daffy and Ian and Smidge. Told you a bit about Daffy, didn't I? Ian and Smidge, they're cousins but they live together with Ian's parents 'cause Smidge's Dad is doing a ten-year stretch and his mam's done a runner with this moron from London. I think it's London anyway. Somewhere down there. Thinks he's dead cool. Shit. Happens all the time – mams going off when the dads get time. Well, not *all* the time but a lot. Couldn't see my mam doing it, though. Not my mam, but there you go. Anyway, thing about Smidge was he was always late for everything. Kept telling him he'd end up being late for his own funeral. Just *couldn't* be on time. Reason I'm telling you that is because *that* afternoon he *was* on time but if he *had* been late like he usually was we wouldn't have been down the front like we were. Now *that's* what you can call fate if you like. It had to be *that* day he was ready in time. Anyway, Daffy had this car, just a

119

banger but it went, and we all piled in and off we went to Sheffield. Left, dunno, *really* early. Seemed like the middle of the night. Really great, it was. Great feeling. This was *big*, you see. Cup semi-final and all. Had to park miles from the ground, I remember. Pigs everywhere. That's police, you know. And then walk. Even when *we* got there and we thought we were going to be early, there were tons of people there already. Can't really tell you about the atmosphere. Just terrific. You'd have to have been there to really understand it. Just terrific. That's all I can say. Seemed like the whole of Liverpool was there. Terrific. Everyone laughing and shouting and taking the mickey out of everyone else. Just a big rave, really. Better. Didn't know then what was going to happen, did we? Jesus, if we had . . . if we had. Shit. Sorry. Scares the shit out of me still. See? Look, see my hands? Can't stop them shaking. Not even now. Makes every bit of me shake when I think about it. No. Don't worry. Used to it now, I am. Don't like thinking about it. You can understand that. Don't like talking about it. Don't *like* talking about it, but I don't mind. Got to sometime, don't I? Might as well be now. Gets it outside me, if you know what I mean. Takes it away a bit. From in here. Clears my head a bit. Until it fills up again, that is. Seems like I can feel it filling up sometimes. Like someone pouring water into it. Pouring memories in from a jug or something. Really weird, it is. I can sometimes be lying there on my bed and with my eyes closed and I can *see* the level going up. First I see my head empty and then there's this stuff getting poured in and the level starts rising. That's when I start to shout at myself. That's what scares Mam – when I start having these shouting fits. Just lying there shouting. What? Oh, dunno. Never know that. Never have a clue *what* it is I'm shouting. Just shouting. Yeah, words, sure, but dunno what words. Can't ever remember and Mam can't make them out so I guess we'll never know. Doesn't matter. No big deal. I can handle it okay. Can't stop it, like, but can handle it. Got to, don't I? Go mad if I couldn't. Know what I used to think? Used to think it was some sort of punishment. Stupid. Dunno. Punishment for what I really don't know. For nothing, probably. Just wanted it to be a punishment for something maybe. I dunno. For living maybe. Like a penance sort of. You Catholic? Okay then, you'll know what I'm at. Tell your sins and do your penance, your five Hail Marys or whatever and everything's fine after that. Bit like that, I think. Dunno. Really don't know. But I don't think I think that any more. Don't think about it at all if I can help it. Just have my shouting fits and get on with things. Treat it like coughing or something. Part of living, that's all. My way of living anyway. Part of my way of living. You've got a right one here, haven't you? Right nutter, I bet you're thinking. Tell you a secret: Mam thinks I've gone in the head. She won't tell *you* that. Or me. But she thinks it all right. Can't say I blame her. Dad? Told you, didn't I? He agrees with Mam so I s'pose he thinks I'm a nutter now, too. Got to laugh, don't you? . . . You know why I'm rabbiting on, don't you? Trying to put off telling you. Guessed that, didn't you? Building myself up to it, like they say. Getting there, too. Soon enough. You can always cut all this crap out anyway, can't you? Edit your tape or whatever. Up to you. Use what you want and dump the rest. Dump the lot if you like. Your choice. Anyway, got to have a pee.

Okay. Ready again. You ready? Got it going? Good. Have it all worked out in my head now. Just have to say it. I won't stop or anything. Just keep going, I will, till I get it all said. Easier for me that way. Okay? Well, the first thing is we all got separated. We were all being funnelled into this one place, the Liverpool fans, I mean, and everyone rushing and shoving to get down the front. And with all the rushing and pushing, we got split up. Just as well, as it turned out, but I was pretty pissed off about it at the time. Like my mates with me. Part of the whole thing, it is, having your mates with you at matches. In case of trouble, too. Need them in case of trouble. Watch your back for you. Anyway, there I was on my tod down the front, about sort of four or five back from the very front. Jesus Christ, it was packed. Talk about your sardines! Worse than that, it was. I had my hands in my anorak pockets and I couldn't get them out. We were that packed. Didn't mind, though. Part of it, wasn't it? Thing I remember best was that you couldn't sort of move at all by yourself. Had to wait for *everyone* to move before you could. Then you *had* to shift even if you didn't want to. Sway like. A lot of swaying. But you get that. No one was worried. Just laughing and carrying on and shouting for the Reds. You should have heard the roar when the teams came on. Couldn't hear the Forest fans. Not with the racket we were making. Terrific . . . Anyway, they said – in the papers and things later – that they'd been playing about six minutes when it

121

happened. Didn't seem like six minutes, though. Seemed like they'd just kicked off, really. Seemed to come from the back. The pushing. No, not pushing. Just a kind of downward sway. Seemed like a bit of a joke at first. We were all still laughing and cheering. S'pose even then some must have been screaming down the very front but you couldn't have heard them. Couldn't have heard them. Not with all the cheering and stuff. Fuck. Still think about that, I do. Them getting crushed to death and us not knowing, probably still laughing and them getting crushed to death like that . . . Anyway, first I knew something was wrong was all those pigs running over and getting a right jeering. Thought it was a fight or something had broken out and the pigs were coming to stop it. Happens. Bound to. Everyone all geed up the way they are. But then the pigs started running about like blue-arsed flies, shouting at one another and looking like they didn't know what to do. One was sort of waving at us to move back. Stupid fucker. How the hell could we move back. Couldn't move at all except down the way we were being pushed. Then the match was stopped and – you know something? – it was like the place went really quiet. It *didn't* go quiet of course, just quieter, and that's when I heard the real screaming for the first time. No. That's not right. That's when I *think* I heard the screaming. Maybe I never heard any screaming at all but I keep telling myself I did. Doesn't matter. Anyway, that's when people started to panic. I know I did. Really shit-scared I got. Found myself sort of not being able to breathe although it could have been the fright that made me feel like that, I suppose. I could see some lads trying to clamber over the fencing and the pigs trying to help them get over – that, for some stupid reason, made it all seem really serious. I mean, the last thing you'd expect was the pigs trying to help people get *on* to the pitch. After that, I dunno. I dunno what really happened. Just felt myself falling forward and couldn't do fuck all about it. Everyone around me was falling forward too. All mixed up. I see things still, in my mind like, but couldn't swear it's what happened. Just sort of pictures. Seems like someone was cutting through the wiring, the fencing like, and everyone was landing up on the pitch. All in a heap, sort of. That's where I found myself anyway. I was on top of this bloke and I said, 'What the fuck's going on?'. And he was staring at me. Just staring at me. I know now he was dead but I didn't know then. Knew something was up with him but, you know something, I couldn't get up off of him. Just couldn't move at all. Wanted to. Could have – I mean, there was nothing holding me there, no one else on top of me – but couldn't make myself move, if that makes any sense. Next thing I know someone is rolling me off of him. Ambulance, I think. Maybe police but I think ambulance, and they were kneeling over him, giving him a good going over and trying to give him the kiss of life and all. I was just sitting there, I think. Not doing anything. Someone did ask me if I was okay and I remember nodding, but all I had in my head was that dead bloke over there on the grass and sort of wondering if I'd done for him. Me lying on top of him and not getting off had done for him. Like a bloody battlefield it was. Know why I say that? 'Cause someone else said it at the time. Dunno who. Someone near me said, 'Jesus, it's like a bloody battlefield'. That sticks in here, in my head. Was worse than that, really. Like you *expect* bodies and all in battle, don't you, but not at a frigging football match. Yeah, I think that's it, too. The sort of surprise of it all. Nobody could *believe* it. I know I kept saying something like 'it's not happening' to myself and I guess others were doing the same. Dunno for sure about that, but I guess they were. Had to be. All you could think, really. It's not happening. But it did. It sure as hell did.

Dunno how I got home. I swear to this day I dunno how I got home. Just arrived, that's all. Mam says I got home and seemed perfectly okay. Told them all about it and all, but I don't remember any of that. Daffy and Midge came round, not Ian, Daffy and Midge only, but I don't remember that either. Don't honestly remember anything till I woke up the next morning. And that was some waking up I can tell you. It was all there bang in my head then. Every little detail. But I couldn't sort of believe it. Not till I saw the papers and telly and stuff. Then I *had* to believe it, didn't I? No getting away from it. Still isn't. Never will be, I think. Stuck with it. Know something? Wanted to find out the name of that lad I'd been on top of. Wanted to go to his funeral. Tried everything, I did, but no one could tell me for sure. Could have been any one of them, you see. That still hurts me a lot. Couldn't go to his funeral. Been with him, hadn't I, when he died. Last person on earth with him. Seemed right to go to his funeral, but I couldn't. Guess it might have been all right if it could have stopped there. No such luck.

123

Sorry. That's not what I mean. Just didn't stop, did it? Not with all the enquiry and everything. Kept reminding me of everything all over again. Got really morbid, I did. Couldn't wait to see it played over and over on the telly. Think I kept trying to see myself. Not just to see myself. Not like those morons who like to see themselves on the telly, waving and all. More like I wanted to be sure I *had* been there although I knew I had been. Dunno why I wanted that. Good one for the old psychiatrist, that one is. I dunno, though.

Funny. Mam says I didn't start getting moody till much later. Not till everything had pretty well died down. Didn't know I was getting moody myself. Thought I was just the same as ever. Until I started ripping down the posters and stuff. Burning them. I knew something was different about me then, all right, but I just put it down to – dunno really – kind of cleaning up, getting ready to start again, I suppose. Don't ask me why I wanted to clean up. Not like me, that isn't. And to burn my collection . . . no explanation for that. Anyway, I never did start again. Couldn't. Can't. Can't stand the whole business of football. Like I said, it's shit now. Football. Shit. For me. Like I'm waiting and waiting and waiting for something to happen again, and more people getting killed for one reason or another, and I sure as anything not wanting to be there and any part of it. Can you blame me? You find yourself lying on someone dead and see what it does to you. Really blows your mind. That's what it does. Me – example number one. Yeah, I know. I know all that. Keep telling myself, don't I, that it's unlikely to happen again. But it might. It just might, mightn't it? And then what? What if something disastrous did happen and I was there stuck in the thick of it again, eh? Want me to really go off my rocker?

Yeah, sure, I know it's just me. I mean, Daffy still goes. So do Midge and Ian but not as much, I think. But that's up to them, isn't it? Me, I've got to deal with little ole me, and there's no way this side of hell you'd get me going again. Or even looking at it. Just don't want to know. Simple as that. Just don't want to know, mate. Keep myself to myself, that's my new motto.

Do? What d'you mean 'do'? Oh. I see. Nothing, I guess. Sit here. Listen to a bit of music. Eat. Sleep. Think. Yeah, I think a lot. Think about the way things used to be. Raves and things we used to go to.

Discos. Pubs. Cinema. Not brooding or anything, you mustn't think that. Just sitting here having thoughts – that's a bit different from thinking, isn't it? I think it is anyway. Lost interest in doing most things but don't mind the thought of them coming into my head. Lost interest in everything, really. Can't think of – if you asked me to name one thing that interested me now, I mean really interested me, I couldn't tell you a single thing. Nothing does. Not now. Just for now. I'll get out of it one day, you see if I don't. Know I will. Got to.

No, haven't seen the lads for ages. Got really pissed off with me, they did. Can't blame them. Can't blame them. Get fed up with myself, I would, if I was them. Not much fun I'm not now. Yeah, they used to be round all the time, watching videos, having a bit of a laugh and stuff. I'm sure Mam asked them to come. To cheer me up. She'd have tried that, okay. Get me to snap out of it. That's the way she puts it. Like some sort of frigging magic – snap your fingers and I snap out of it as if I was hypnotised or something. But like I said, they got pissed off with trying to make me cheery. Got to get on with their own lives, haven't they? Can't just waste their time on me. Anyway, to tell you the honest truth, don't want them around no more. Don't want anyone round. Just want me around me. Mam says I'm selfish, but I don't see it that way. I think I'm generous. Not wanting to waste anyone's time or sympathy. That's something else – I'll strangle the next fucker who starts off with that sympathy bit, going all mushy when they're talking to me like I was a baby in a buggy or a halfwit or something like that. Good job you didn't try that sort of approach – but you wouldn't, would you? I can see that.

So there you are, mate. That's the sad tale of Brendan Keyes. Makes you weep, don't it? Makes you laugh, more like. Got to frigging laugh. Got to. I do when I'm alone. Sure, cry too, but laugh as well. Don't know why and don't care. Enough on my plate without having to figure all that stuff out. Quite enough. Quite enough to cope with for a while. For ever maybe. Who knows? Who fucking cares?

The last information I had on Brendan came in a letter from his mother. She felt he was making headway, improving slightly, now that she had succeeded in getting him to have regular consultations with a woman psychologist. I hope his progress continues.

125

ELEVEN

Wicked, isn't it, your own dad

TOM LIVINGSTON

Tom Livingston is twenty-two, slightly built, five foot six, with very dark curly hair. Because his hair flops about his eyes he has developed a quirk of tossing his head even when his hair is in place. His eyes are large, wide-set and deep blue. He is extremely handsome, and knows it, but not in any arrogant way. He jokes about it. 'Can't go past a mirror without having a bit of a preen,' he says. 'All that's left to me is my looks, so why not let myself enjoy them, eh?'

Tom lives with his adoptive parents in Southampton. He was fostered to them when he was thirteen, officially adopted when he was sixteen. At the age of nine he was taken into care when it was suspected he was being sexually abused by his natural father, although no charges were ever brought.

Tom's hobby is writing to pen-friends. He has some twenty of these, in all parts of the world. He writes an excellent letter and it was through one of these that he contacted me. Since coming to live in Scotland I have done what small bit I can to help youngsters coming out of care, and it was based on their experiences that I wrote my novel *Skating Round the Poppy.* Tom read this novel and wrote to me to say it was 'pretty good'. I sent him a postcard thanking him for his note. By return I had another letter from him in which he went into more detail in his criticism, and it wasn't difficult to tell that he had been through the same abuse that many of these youngsters have had to bear. We wrote back and forth several times, and in one of my letters I told him that I was writing this book. He said he would like to talk to me, 'to put me straight', making it clear that his parents had said it would be all right.

From much of what he said in his letters I suspected that Tom might indeed be a victim of post traumatic stress, and it was on this basis that I agreed to come south and visit him.

When I arrived at his home Tom was out, and his parents took the opportunity to tell me that they did not think Tom was completely over his experiences. He was, they said, making 'giant strides', but that he was given to flashes of almost uncontrollable anger, often leading to violence which erupted without warning, usually when he had been in a state of excitement. They warned me he was excited about my visit and that should he become angry while talking to me, all I needed to do was sit still and wait quietly until the anger subsided. They advised me it would be unwise to argue with him. When Tom came home ('Been down the shops to get some fags to keep the nerves steady'), it was hard to believe that he could be violent. He appeared to be a perfectly normal twenty-two-year-old. He was polite and witty, eager to take me up to his room and talk.

Bet they told you all about me, didn't they? No? Bet they did. Said they would. Told me they would. That's really why I went out. Had fags here all the time. Wanted to let them have a chat with you. Fill you in, like. Easier that way, coming from them. Thought you'd believe them more. No, I'm not going to lie to you. Why should I? But some things are better coming from someone else. You know the way it is. Me telling you about myself might not be that exact. Everyone changes the facts a bit when they're admitting to faults, don't they? Any sort of faults. Even ones you can't help. Can't control, sort of. Natural, really. Sort of protection. That thing picking all this up? Better be careful then, hadn't I? Might incriminate myself. Joke. Just a joke. You wouldn't be here if I didn't trust you. Promise you that. Funny. Feel like I know you pretty well. From that book. Funny how a book can make you feel you know the bloke who wrote it. Don't, of course. Don't know you at all. Know the way you think, though. And that's important. If what you said in the book was meant. If it was all bullshit then I'm in trouble. Got to take a chance on you, though. That's what I'm doing really: taking a chance on you. Let me down and you're dead meat. Don't really mean that. Be hurt, I will. Hurt. They tell you I could get pretty violent? Thought so. Good. That's fine. Wanted them to. Better to know these things to begin with. Hope I won't be. Don't expect I will. No reason. Don't always need a reason, though. Well, what I mean is *I* have a reason or think I do, but often it's not a real reason. I know that. I'm aware of that. Just can't do nothing about it. Just happens. Soon calm down, though. And forget all about it. That's the good thing, I think. That I forget about it. And they do, too, so everyone's happy in the end. Happy ever after. Everyone has their ups and downs, don't they? Like people get sad and happy and angry, don't they. That's how it is with me, only I go way over the top. Like when I get sad I get depressed, and when I get happy I get too happy, hysterical almost, and when I get angry I blow my top and get violent. Just my way. I know all about it, you see. Just got to find a way of controlling it all. Controlling my emotions. Easier said than done, though. But I'm coming along. Much better than I used to be. They'll tell you that. Do it for them, really. Want them to be happy. Great, they are. Put up with all sorts of shit from me they have. Surprised they haven't chucked me out years ago. I would have. Chucked myself out, I mean. Rotten bastard I've been sometimes. Sometimes *wanting* to hurt them, and that's not right. That's *all* wrong. Getting back at myself, I think. Or someone. Don't rightly know. Anyway, like I told you, I'm getting better at controlling things now. Much better. Quite chuffed with myself, I am, when I think about it. Yeah, sure, sure I think about it. Don't always make much sense out of it, though. Some sense but not much. Like after I've exploded over something I'll come up here and have a think about it. It's called rationalising. Know that? Anyway, that's what I try and do – rationalise. Sometimes it works, sometimes it don't. If it does it does, if it don't it don't. Nothing I can do about it. Way the head works. That's when it works at all. Sometimes it goes on strike. Pickets out and all. Just blank. Nothing. Blank. Zero. Zilch. That's the worst. Find myself hitting my head with my fists sometimes, trying to wake it up. Knock some sense into it. Make it function. Get those little grey cells working. Ha – watch that too, do you? Crap really, isn't it. Stupid old

129

fart he is, that Poirot. Little grey cells my arse. Don't like grey. Red or green or blue. That'd be better. More alive, don't you think? More alert, anyway. That's what I think. The way I see it.

Better get down to the basics, hadn't we? Didn't come all this way to hear me talking about stupid coloured cells. Be a laugh that though, wouldn't it? Coming all the way down here and end up with just that? I know *you* wouldn't think it funny, but it'd be a laugh just the same. Okay. Down to basics. Only way to do it is to come out and say it. That's what I find. I'll do that. Do it now. You know why I was put into care, don't you? I did tell you, didn't I? Can't remember. Can't remember half of what I said in my letters. You know anyway? Okay. Abused. That's really a laugh. Was fucked, I was. For years. By my dad. My real dad. Wicked, that is, isn't it? Your own dad doing that to you. Bad enough someone else, someone you don't really know, but your own dad – what's wicked. Evil, really. Like who can you trust if you can't trust your dad? Answer me that. No one, that's who. And then he does this to you and you're all fucked up in the head. And you can't really hate him for it, can you? You can't go round hating your dad. That's another part of it. The worst part maybe. Knowing he's a bastard and a shit and still you can't hate him. Got to keep on loving him even after what he's done. Even start making excuses for him, you do. Like, well, my mum was a right slag. Always drunk and knocking off with other men. And she'd mock him – my dad. In front of us kids, me and my sister. Think she was my sister, anyway. Was always told she was but she didn't look nothing like us. Anyway, she'd say stuff like 'If you were a proper man I wouldn't have to' – stuff like that. And I'd use that sometimes and tell myself that's why he was doing it to me. Bit like the bloke in your book he was. Always being nice about it. Never really threatening me or anything. Just telling me he loved me. That was pretty important to me – being loved. I guess he sussed that and used it. Wasn't getting any off my mum, was I? She didn't give a monkey's about me. In the way, I was. So, like, I *had* to sort of hang on to what I was getting from my dad. And he used that. I can see that now. Sure I can. He was really using that. But in a kind of way I suppose I thought something was better than nothing. When you've got nothing, *anything* is better, isn't it? I think so. Or thought so at the time anyway. Even now, even now when I go through it – huh? Yes. All the time. Keep going through it. Can't shake it, can I? – anyway, when I go through it the thing I think of most is him saying he loved me and I keep wondering that maybe he *did* love me, so how can I hate him? Wish I could. Wish to fuck I could. Be easy then. Dead easy. Could rub it all out. Think I could, anyway. Never know, though, 'cause I can't hate him. Yes, that's for sure, I really hated what he was doing to me, but that's different. Kind of like I could separate what he was doing from him. Hated it but didn't hate him. Stupid, isn't it, when you come to think about it. Should be able to link the two but can't. Like having two different people, really. One doing it and one loving you. Different people.

Worst day of my life when they took me away and put me into care. All I did was cry. Still do when I think about it. When I'm alone and think about it. Awful, it was. Just fucking awful. All confusing. Like I was pleased he couldn't get at me any more but with him not with me I'd no one to say they loved me. Go on about that, don't I? Must have been important to me. Someone loving me. Insecure, I suppose. And then, in this way I was all feeling guilty – like I'd let *him*, my dad, down. Explain it? Can't. Don't think I can. Try if you like. Well, let's have a think . . . Okay. This is going to sound real messy. Stupid. Best I can do, though. You really want to hear it? Okay. Lots of things come into it. Like I'd be in my bed and I'd be thinking of my mum having a go at him and I'd see him all buckled up and sort of afraid of her. Don't think he *was* afraid of her, but I'd see him that way. That was one thing. Didn't like to think of him like that at all. Then – let's see – well, I *missed* him. He could be great too. Taking me places and having fun. Took me to this circus once. Brilliant. And I suppose because I missed him I felt he would be missing me. Like I'd let him down. I told you it would be messy. Understand what I'm saying? Good. 'Cause I don't. Not really. I mean I know I couldn't have done anything about them taking me away but I still sort of feel I should have done something. Dunno what. Something. And, look, just suppose, I'd think, suppose he *did* really love me, what was he going to do now? All that sort of thing. That's what made me feel kind of guilty. Anyway, I'm stopping for now. You go down and Mum will give you something. Tea, I think. I know she got some cake this morning so

131

you'll get that too if you're lucky. I need a break. Go on, piss off for now.

Should apologise, shouldn't I? Yes I should. Know I should. Shouldn't have told you to piss off. Did you a favour really if you want to know. Was getting tight in here. Going to have a go at you, I think. Know I was. Better to get you out of the way. Part of what I told you – starting to control things. Year ago and I *would* have had a go at you. A right go, probably. Used to do that all the time. Just lash out. Still do a bit. Not often. Not as often as I did, but a bit. Like when I go for a drink. Do that. Drink. Nothing that you'd call much. But even one pint'll get me going. Be standing there minding my business and someone'll say something to me, something quite nice and friendly probably, and bingo, I'll hit him. Feel sorry afterwards. Always do. Always feel sorry. But what's the good of being sorry when you've done it. Should feel sorry *before* you do it. That'd be the right thing. Sensible thing. That's what I'm trying to teach myself. Feel sorry first. Save all the aggro, that would. But I don't seem able to think that way. Not yet. Not when the situation comes up. Anyway, where were we?

Yeah, I sure did. For ages. Years. Thought I might be queer. Like what he did to me had made me queer. Didn't fancy men or anything. Used to make myself sick thinking of going with a man, but that didn't stop me thinking I might be that way. Made me really aggressive towards the queers too. Didn't go out bashing them or anything, don't think that, but I'd always have a good verbal at them when I saw them. Loads around here. Hunting the sailors and things. Loads. Think I thought that if I had a go at them I'd be protecting myself. Like if I *was* queer I wouldn't slag them off, would I? So when I did it it was like proving to myself I wasn't. That make any sense? Yeah, I've had girls. Nothing serious. Can't seem to keep one for long. Tell myself love 'em and leave 'em, but that's just fooling myself. I know that. Just can't seem to keep the thing going no matter how much I like them or want them. Soon as they get too close, too serious about it all, I drop them. Don't want to drop them, mind. Just do it, and end up feeling sorry for myself. Get over that one by telling myself they didn't deserve me. Good, eh? Amazing what you can kid yourself into believing if you put your mind

132

to it. Same with friends. Can't hold on to them. Don't even have to have a row with them. Just – like – suddenly, something makes me cancel them. Doesn't have to be a reason. I want them and I don't want them, if you can understand that. Just come back here and feel sorry for myself and then I'll blow up. Smash things. Done that too. Smashed things. Things I like. Smashed my stereo once. Really pissed me off, that did, when I seen what I'd done. Getting better at that, too. More discriminating. That's a good word. Discriminating. Can't be all that stupid, can I? Like I only smash things that I don't really care about now, so I must be putting some sort of thought into it even if I am acting crazy.

No, not what you'd really call lonely. Alone, sure. But not lonely. Don't think I get lonely, anyway. Never sat down and said to myself 'you're lonely'. Go really round the bend if I got into that. Just don't want people round me. Too suspicious, I think. Suspicious of everyone. Wondering what they're up to, what they want, what they're after. I can tell myself they're not after anything but I don't really believe it. Like I'm lying to myself. That's maybe why I cancel my friends. It's a bit as though because I do really like them that I cancel them – so that I don't find out they're after something. I want to keep liking them even though they're not my friends any more. Even at work – got me this job in the market – even there I don't mix in much. Just do my job and whizz off home. Don't fight or anything, don't get me wrong, just don't mix. Better all round. Get too close to anyone and I know there'll be a falling out. My fault. Don't want to cause hassle at work. Need the job. So, like I says, do my job and off back home.

Naw, can't see it. Can't see myself ever getting married. Like to. Love to. Love to have kids and treat them really well. Protect them from all the shit that goes on. But I can't see it. Nobody'd have me – that's bullshit. Just looking for – you know – you to tell me there'd be lots girls to have me – flatter me sort of, make me feel good – and you'd be right, even if I do say so myself. No point in giving myself crap. I know I'm better looking than most. Been told it often enough. Better looking than all those wankers that are supposed to be sex symbols, ain't I? And there *are* lots of birds who'd go out with me if I asked them, and maybe even marry me. But it would never last. Not in a million years. I'd see to that. I'd ruin it. Can't do that to a woman, can you? Not right.

Mucking up her life and maybe even the kids' life if we had any. Shouldn't ever do that to kids. Have them trust you and feel secure and then just go off and leave them. And that's what I would do. Go off. Know I would. Yeah, I know I would. I do know it. And then where'd I be, tell me that? I'd really have some guilt on my shoulders then, wouldn't I? Like the hunchback of wherever it is. Yes. Notre Dame. Okay, dam. Couldn't handle that at all. No, what I think I'll have to do is stay a – ha, nearly said 'a bachelor gay', but you can't say that now, can you? Have people talking. Stay a confirmed bachelor, that's another way they put it, isn't it? Leave all those lovely birds craving for me – I don't fucking think! Still, might be one or two who would still be wanting me. Nice sort of thought, that. Really love myself, don't I? Shit, mate, can't stand myself if you really want the truth, the whole truth and nothing but the truth, so help me God. Too busy He is. Up to His eyes. No help coming from that quarter. Like the way I look and all, but the inside of me I can't stand. No point in trying to con myself about that. Or trying to. Have tried. Got nowhere, though. Won't till I get everything sorted out and shit knows how long that's going to take. For ever. And that means never, doesn't it. End of story.

Yeah. Sure. I'll go on writing to you if that's what you want. Pleased to. My pleasure. Didn't think you'd want me to. Why? Dunno. Just didn't think you'd be interested. Can't be very interesting for you. Not what I write. You really want me to? Okay. No problem . . . Listen – no. Forget it. Stupid . . . Okay. Look, you remember in one of your letters you said something about me maybe coming up to stay with you for a few days and meeting those other lads you know who – you know – had done to them what I had? You mean that? You're sure? Wasn't just you saying it to be kind or something? Okay. Thanks. Okay. Dunno, do I? Have to think about that one. Probably not. Could say no now. Definitely no . . . Yeah, okay, you're right. I *do* want to come up but I'm not going to tell you that, am I? Put a bad sign on it if I did that. Got to pretend I *don't* want to. That way it might just work out all right. See you.

Tom does still write to me, once a fortnight with great regularity. His letters are long and chatty. He has not, thus far, made any reference to our

134

conversation apart from enquiring when 'that book's going to be in the shops'. Indeed, he says less now about himself than he did prior to the interview. For my part, I have also avoided making any reference to our talk. I feel sure he will bring it up eventually, when he feels the time is right.

Happily, in his last but one letter, he intimated that he might come up and visit me.

TWELVE

An everlasting limbo

GERHART LECHNER

Gerhart Lechner is sixty-two and lives in south-west London. He is a small man but very broad, as wide as he is tall, as they say. Everything about him, apart from his voice, gives the impression of ferocity. He has a mop of unruly grey hair, thick bushy eyebrows that meet over the bridge of his nose, and his eyes, grey, stare at you discomfortingly when he speaks to you. Yet his voice, although heavily accented, is deep and kind, soothing.

It is ironic that of all the people I interviewed he was the only one who said I could use his own name. Gerhart Lechner is not his real name although it is the one he has grown up with and used nearly all his life. He does not know his real name. It was stolen from him. Just as he was stolen from his parents.

Gerhart Lechner was born and spent the first six years of his life somewhere in western Poland. That is all he knows. Following the German invasion of his country it became Nazi policy to requisition all Aryan children – particularly the blue-eyed, fair-haired ones – and transport them to Germany for what they called 'Germanisation'. The man in charge of this 're-stocking' of the German nation with true Aryan types was Heinrich Himmler. Shortly before his sixth birthday Gerhart Lechner was one of fifty children thus taken and sent by train to a

Germanisation centre. He was given the name Gerhart Lechner and all other information about him was destroyed.

Yes. You would think that. You would think that after more than half a century the pain would ease, that you could forget, that you would, perhaps, no longer wish to know, that you would not care. But it is not so, my friend. It is indeed not so. Certainly, yes, you do forget certain things. Details, yet other details grow in your mind and transfix you on occasions. There is a word: loom. That is the word to use. They loom. The image of the morning we were put on the train looms. Like it was, quite truly, yesterday. I could tell you every detail. What I wore. What my mother was wearing. What the weather was like. The smells. Everything. Yes, they did that. They brought our mothers to the station. It made us easier to control. That was what they had worked out. But not on to the platform. My mother, with all the others, was kept back behind a high wire fence while we were loaded on to the train. I can see her still. I can hear her. She is calling my name. And that is the source of my biggest nightmare. Still. She is calling my name and I cannot hear that name because of the din the other mothers are making. Calling the names of their children. If I could just hear what she was calling. Just hear my name . . .

Our first stop was an assessment and selection centre. They were very thorough. Everything about us was examined. Eyes, ears, lips, noses, shape of head. Limbs measured. Colour of hair. Two things you must remember. Firstly, we were to be Germans so we had to be racially perfect. Secondly, since we were – in their estimation – only Poles, if we did not measure up, if we failed in the smallest detail, we were expendable. Many children did fail. It could be anything. Eyes were very important. Those with dark eyes had far less chance of being selected than those, like myself, with blue eyes. Even those who did not stand up straight could be put aside. That was the way it was. Germans stood up straight. Slavs, for example, hunched their shoulders. That is what was said. Those who failed? Ah. They were sent to concentration camps to die. Far more were rejected than were selected. We were told that. To make those of us selected feel more important, I should say. The start of the Germanisation. The arrogance that was needed. Our superiority over the sub-humans. I still remember that, and remember that, to my shame, I *was* proud to be selected. It was a terrible thing to do to a child.

In any case, armed with our new names and our new identities, those of us who were selected were sent to camps set aside for the Nazi Youth. Four of us went to my camp. We were forbidden then to speak Polish. We were forbidden to play with each other. We had to speak German and play with the German children. I know that sounds cruel. It *was* cruel, of course, but even then, already, after such a short time, I was having those feelings of – can I say it? – Germany? It now saddens me but I must say that I enjoyed those times in the Nazi Youth camp. They were good days for children. What child would not enjoy them? Swimming and football and orienteering? Even the uniforms we wore gave us – how can I put it – a sense of pride, however false that pride might have been. Forget? No, I never *forgot* that I was Polish, but . . . Well, you must understand the times. Poles, you see, were *untermensch*, racially well below the Germans. They were used as labourers. We would see lines of them going and coming from work. Dirty and cowered. What child would like to be like that? A child doesn't think in terms of patriotism. No, that is not true. I think a child does. But given the chance, as we were, a child would always, I think, opt to be patriotic to the country that made him feel – yes, superior. A child, even the most loved child, is filled with doubts and insecurities, is he not? How, then, could I expect myself to choose to belong to the race that did all the menial work? I could not. In particular since I was already believing that I was superior in every way to them. We were all so impressionable. We did not want to – to lose our new friendships. Don't forget these were all German boys. Hitler was their idol. He became my idol. I admit that freely. We – yes, it is true – we adored Hitler. *Gott!* Six million Poles, my countrymen, were killed on the orders of that man, and I adored him!

Assimilation had to be complete, total. I had to have a German family. I was sent for adoption. It will tell you how methodical, how well-planned the entire operation was that the family I was sent to was the Lechners. I had been given the name over a year earlier, so the family I was to go to had been already selected. They lived in Köln – Cologne.

Kind people. Very kind. Childless. They worshipped me. Gave me everything I wanted. My father – and that is how I still think of him – was an engineer with Mercedes Benz. A very proud man. Very proud to be German and he did much to instill that pride in me. That, I know now, was why he had chosen to be the father of one of us Polish-born children. When Germany lost the war, it killed him. Not physically. He lived for many years. But he wilted. Shrivelled up. Died. He was never the same. And his being like that killed my new mother. Literally. She died in nineteen-fifty. For no reason. From no ailment other than seeing her husband wasting away. It was very sad. For me, too, since I did love them. I might have misled you by calling Mutti my 'new' mother. She was, you see, simply my mother. In truth, all memory of my *real* mother had been eradicated at that time. I truly, by that stage, believed I was German and that these two kind people were my parents. I probably believed it because I *wanted* to believe it. The reason doesn't really matter. The simple fact is that I *did* believe it. And even that is not the truth. In here, in my heart, I was German, but in here, in my brain, hidden away so I never thought about it, I was still Polish. And just sometimes, oh, very seldom, something would happen, someone would say something, or I'd catch the scent of something, or see something, some small thing, and a fragment of that memory would come back, the memory of my very early childhood. But I'd stop it. Instantly. Terrible. Quite terrible. A terrible denial, but I was so young. Only nineteen when Mutti died. Until my father told me. That was the moment, you know, when the box opened within my brain. The moment the real agony began. I was so angry with him. I shouldn't have been. It wasn't me he was trying to hurt. It was himself. He loved me so much, you see, that he thought he had failed me. It was himself he wanted to hurt. I have never seen such fury in a man's eyes as he screamed at me, 'Yes, yes, you are a damned Pole!'.

You will appreciate that after the war there was considerable turmoil and chaos. Quite apart from the liberation of those in the concentration camps, Germany was a land of displaced persons. A land of total uncertainty. Many wished to return to their homelands but were afraid to do so; so much territory was now occupied by the Russians, and rumours abounded about their treatment of people. I think the only security I had at the time was in the misplaced knowledge that I was German. That I had a country. But I didn't. I could, perhaps, have continued to *believe* I had, had not my father . . . as I told you.

It is difficult to explain, to enumerate all the emotions. I certainly cannot put into words the horror . . . true horror I felt at hearing my father's words. Not only the words themselves but the way he said them. The hatred in his voice. It was as though, when I thought, when I *knew* he loved me, he was telling me he hated me. And then there was the inexplicable guilt I felt. Guilt at denying I was Polish if, indeed, I was Polish. And if I was, what of my real parents? I had never, it seemed to me, given them a thought. Not cared what had happened to them. Denied, in a way, their existence. Can you understand what I'm saying? Can you understand at all what that did to me? What I'm saying is I had spent those years being someone I wasn't, being a citizen of a country that wasn't mine, that had stolen me, giving my love to parents who were not my parents, who had participated in the deception. So now I had to ask myself, who am I? I didn't *want* to be anyone else. I wanted to be the person I was, but I could not, could I, since that person was a fraud, a fake. That person was *not* a person. It was just a false name. Nothing more. A name with no one to go with it. Do I make sense?

Why? Ah, yes. I am sorry. I should have explained. After the war a Polish Resettlement Office was set up in Berlin. West Berlin. Somehow they heard about me. Through one of the other children who had been taken from Poland at the same time I was, I think. I don't know. But I think I recall hearing something like that. It would be natural. Everyone presumed, you see, that we – all the children who had been stolen, that is – would be unhappy and anxious to get back to our real parents if they were still alive. So, someone probably thought they were doing me a kindness. Anyway, two people came to the house, my father's house. My father was out. They asked me questions about myself. It was frightening. They asked me if I was one of the stolen children, and I said, I said . . . I said, no. I showed them my papers, the German papers that had been made out for me shortly after I was taken to Germany. They showed my name and showed where I had been born, in Köln, and that I was the son of my father, Hans Lechner. It was all quite friendly. They explained everything and apologised for coming. I remember the relief and my thinking that if they were

141

convinced then I must be who I was. Then my father came in. Something had happened to him that day – I never discovered what – but he was very upset, very agitated when he came in. He demanded, quite angrily, out of character completely, who these strangers were. I told him, and made a joke out of why they had come. It was then that he said – what he said. Yes. That was how it came about. And from that moment I was two things: I was a nobody and a very different human being. It was as though not only my identity had been taken from me, but my mind too, my reason. My ability to reason anyway.

And so, my friend, so started my life of – my life of what I call the everlasting limbo. I left my home and for some years just wandered throughout Germany. There was nothing extraordinary in this. Germany was a land of nomads. Everyone seeking lost loved ones, seeking to get back to their countries of origin, seeking anything – quite a few seeking revenge, and who can blame them. My father? When I left? No. No, he gave no sign of sorrow. He was fatalistic about it. I told him, of course, that I was leaving. He nodded. Didn't even look up at me. Just nodded his head in a weary way as though he had known all along that it would come to this. I wanted so much to embrace him before I left. Perhaps he wanted me to also. I don't know. I will never know. But I couldn't. I was too afraid he would draw back from me and that I would see that terrible hatred in his eyes again. And the extraordinary thing is this: when I heard he had died, I felt no sadness. Just relief. That has always shocked me. Just relief. I cannot understand that.

Oh, after a few years, I think. That would be about right. After two or three years. That was when I found the courage to try and seek my real parents. I sometimes wish I had never started the search. As I know now it was to lead nowhere and it is that vacuum which has given me this awful feeling of isolation. To be truthful, at the start it was a half-hearted effort. It was difficult for me to go to Poland: it was in Russian hands and they were reluctant to let anyone leave. Even those who went on a temporary visa found it difficult to leave. And, anyway, I kept telling myself I had nowhere to start. This was true, certainly, but I could have made the effort. Many people did, and some were rewarded, but most found that their loved ones had died in concentration camps. I wanted to spare myself that discovery. That would have been too much, I think – to have denied the existence of your parents for so long and then find out that they had been murdered. Yes. Yes. Murdered without the comfort of knowing that at least their son would grieve. Oh, yes, I see that now. I see that they might have been alive. But – but – well, even still I did not truly *want* them to be alive. Isn't that shocking? I only hope you will appreciate the confusion that was happening inside me. I don't expect you to. I don't expect anyone to. And I could have contacted the Polish Resettlement Office, but I didn't. I was *afraid*, you see. Afraid of, yes, yes, of being proved to be Polish and sent back. I didn't *want* to go back. I spoke no Polish. And I now thought like a German. I *was*, in fact, a German. I didn't want to be a stranger. Hah. I was a stranger to myself – why would I want to be a stranger to others also? No. No. I didn't want to be Polish. And yet. And yet . . . *denial* is a wicked sin, is it not? A wicked sin.

Dreams? I do not know what it would be like to sleep without them. They are my comfort. How do you say – cold comfort? Yes. Cold comfort, but better than no comfort. I can use them, you see, to pretend it is all a dream. But then, sometimes, less now, but still frequently enough, some small picture will appear in my mind, and I will know it is not a dream. My mother calling my name – that inaudible name. I see that and I know it *did* happen. Someone will light up a strong cigarette and the odour will reach me, and somewhere in the back of my mind I will see, very vaguely, a shadow really, a man lighting such a cigarette, and I will wonder who that man is. My real father? Possibly. Sometimes I see an old metal hoop slung from a tree by a rope. There is a child swinging on it. Someone – sometimes a man, sometimes a woman, is pushing the child. They are laughing. They are happy. And I wonder is that child me and is the person pushing me a parent? I do not know. Or again, someone will be wearing something. You know how it is now – the young girls are taking to wearing old-fashioned clothes? It might be anything – a scarf, a beret, the hair might be tied back with a certain ribbon in a certain style – and again I will see someone in that misty way and wonder if *that* is my mother. Maybe even a sister, if I had one. I do not know.

Oh, yes. Yes, I have really tried in the last ten years. But it is too late now. Records have long since been destroyed. My parents would, I think, certainly be dead by now. Some years ago I spent some months in Poland. Travelling. Everywhere. Trying to see if something, somewhere, would bring something to mind. But nothing did. Although – no, it is silly. It was because I wanted it, you see. I thought once, this might be my birthplace. A pretty place. Very small and peaceful. I half-expected the villagers to rush out and recognise me and call me by my name and embrace me and say, where have you been, we have been waiting so long for you. Very silly. Another dream, you see. A waking dream, may I say that? No, it is too late. Much too late now.

And so I must make the best of what I have. You know, I will be truthful, even now, old man that I am, I still cry at night sometimes, curl myself up in my bed and cry. And suddenly I will shout, Who am I? And then I will be afraid in case someone has heard and I will pull the blankets up over my head, and cry again. That is why I accumulate nothing. I do not like possessions. I do like beautiful things but I will not own them. I cannot. What would become of them? How can I make a will? True, yes, it is true, legally I can make a will, but how can Gerhart Lechner make a will when Gerhart Lechner doesn't exist? And what, when I die, will they put on my gravestone? Must that be a lie also? 'Gerhart Lechner Lies Here'. He doesn't. He never will. No. It is something I must attend to. I must see to it that – never mind. I will deal with that.

May I just tell you one other thing? It is the thing that makes me feel such awful guilt. Why must I tell you? To be honest. With you. With myself. That is why. Sometimes I will see my German mother, my Mutti, and I will run to her with my arms stretched out in front of me and she will be reaching out, saying, come to Mutti, come to Mutti, but as I get closer to her I will hear myself calling Mamusiu, Mamusiu, and then she will start to drift away, to fade, to withdraw from me and her face is no longer filled with joy but with sadness and pain, and I cannot reach her. Mamusiu. Yes. Mamusiu. That is my punishment, my friend. And now you know everything.

A month after I had transcribed this interview I tried to contact Gerhart Lechner. The telephone line was disconnected. I called round to his flat the next time I was in London, only to find that it had been vacated. A week before Christmas I had a letter from Gerhart. It has been written in Warsaw. It was brief. It said simply that he had decided to go and live there. He concluded, 'My health has been poor for some time now, my friend, and this would seem the proper place to die'.

Post Traumatic Stress Disorder

The most common trauma involves serious threat to life or physical integrity, or the sudden destruction of home or community. The disorder is likely to be more deep-seated, and to last longer, when the stress has been caused by human agency. Obviously warfare is such an agency, but other events are less obvious yet equally damaging. In *all* such events the characteristic symptoms involve a re-experiencing of the event and the avoidance of stimuli associated with it, or the numbing of general responsiveness and increased arousal. This may be translated into the following emotive responses:

MEMORIES   reliving combat situations and emotions, remembering lost friends and colleagues, recurring bad dreams.

DISTRESS   when reminded of events because of media coverage, anniversaries, sounds, smells, or sights.

NUMBING   reduced interest in previously significant or pleasurable activities and relationships.

AROUSAL   more irritable and jumpy than usual, and physical signs of tension such as headaches, muscular pains, palpitations and sleep disturbance.

AVOIDANCE   avoiding activities that remind of the traumatic event.

LOSS OF   feeling that emotions may get out of control, and that
  CONTROL   breakdown is imminent.

ANGER   at whatever happened, or at whoever caused it or allowed it; at the injustice and senselessness of it all; at the shame and indignities; at the lack of understanding by others; at the inefficiency of others; directed at innocent individuals such as family, friends, workmates.

GUILT   for surviving when others did not; regret for things not done, or opportunities not taken.

SHAME   for having been exposed as helpless, emotional, and in need of help; for not having acted as one would have wished.

SADNESS   feeling low and prone to weep for deaths, injuries and losses of any kind.

All the above feelings are common, or normal, for anyone who has been through a traumatic experience, be it combat, personal injury, or bereavement. The intensity and number of these feelings varies from person to person, but there are also associated features and complications which can occur in addition to the prime features listed above, and these can make the sufferer very difficult to live with, and lead to marital breakdown and total family disruption.

ANXIETY   over real or imagined situations; may develop into anxiety neurosis, i.e. anxiety over things that only *might* happen.

DEPRESSION   may develop into a major depressive illness.

IMPULSION   appears as a sudden change in life-style and causes the sufferer to, for example, overspend. This has been

148

particularly noticeable among the younger soldiers returning from the Gulf, among the suddenly unemployed with redundancy cheques, and some with criminal injury compensation cheques.

ABUSE the 'I don't care' attitude often leading to self-destructive risk-taking; the physical abuse of others; increased cigarette-smoking and, in the majority of cases, alcohol and/or drug abuse.

SURVIVOR guilt that the sufferer survived when others did not;
GUILT unfounded fear that the sufferer is somehow responsible; may even include sympathy towards the role of the aggressor (Stockholm Syndrome).

PHYSICAL stomach aches, headaches and, in some severe cases,
COMPLAINTS temporary paralysis of limbs.

The above, as already stated, are the emotive responses. However, in examining the PTSD victim, one also has to take into consideration, in relation to the victim's condition:

(1) pre-existing pathology (physical and psychological);
(2) previous exposure to trauma;
(3) life-style and health style;
(4) cultural and ethnic customs;
(5) occupational culture and sub-culture occupations;
(6) pseudo-PTSD;
(7) occupational health (physical and psychological);
(8) criminal and civil breaches or proceedings;
(9) age;
(10) religion;
(11) training;
(12) neuropsychology;
(13) neurophysiology;
(14) disability and special needs.

Legal Report on Zeebrugge Survivors

The process of evaluating victims produces serious problems for both the medical and legal professions when trying to find common ground for treatment and compensation. The following report is a good example. It appeared in the *Independent* and was written by the barrister Shiranikha Herbert.

ZEEBRUGGE SURVIVORS GAIN SHOCK DAMAGES
Arbitration
Re the *Herald of Free Enterprise*.
Before Sir Michael Ogden QC,
      Michael Wright QC,
      William Crowther QC.
February 1989.

A person claiming damages for nervous shock must establish that he is suffering more than grief, distress or other normal human emotion. However, Post Traumatic Stress Disorder and 'pathological grief' which is in excess of normal grief, are recognised psychiatric illnesses for which compensation can be awarded.

It is reasonable for survivors of a disaster to refuse to undergo

151

psychiatric treatment which involves recollecting the circumstances of the disaster.

THE FACTS

The claimants were survivors on the *Herald of Free Enterprise* which capsized off Zeebrugge, Belgium, on 6 March 1987. Under a compensation agreement the survivors received fixed payments of £5,000 each for having been involved in and witnessed the disaster and £5,000 for each relative lost. Under the Fatal Accidents Acts there were fixed payments of £5,000 to the personal representatives for each deceased passenger and a further £5,000 to the estate of the deceased passenger for pre-death injury, pain and suffering in addition to the usual claims for the dependant.

The parties were unable to agree levels of damages for 'nervous shock' which, it was conceded, all the claimants suffered. Ten selected cases went to arbitration.

THE DECISION

The arbitrators said that 'nervous shock' was an odd legal phrase and did not connote shock in the sense often used in ordinary conversation. Lord Bridge said in McLoughlin v O'Brien (1983) AC 410,421 that the common law gave no damages for emotional distress which any normal person experienced when someone he loved was killed or injured. Anxiety and depression were normal human emotions. Yet an anxiety neurosis or a reactive depression might be a recognisable psychiatric illness, with or without psychosomatic symptoms. A claimant had to 'establish that he is suffering not merely grief, distress or any other normal human emotion, but a positive psychiatric illness'.

Post Traumatic Stress Disorder (PTSD) is now a recognised psychiatric illness of the type known as anxiety neurosis. Its essential feature is the development of characteristic symptoms following a psychologically distressing event which is outside the range of usual human experience and which would be distressing to almost anyone. The traumatic event is persistently relived in nightmares and flashbacks, and there is intense distress at exposure to events resembling or symbolising the event. There are also other psychological symptoms.

152

Many Zeebrugge victims suffered PTSD and some suffered other psychiatric illnesses such as depression at the same time. Abnormal or pathological grief was also a common diagnosis among those bereaved, and it was common ground that the circumstances of the bereavement could be significant in determining whether the subsequent grief would be pathological or normal. A person who lost a relative in a horrific circumstance was more likely to suffer pathological grief than if the death was in more normal circumstances.

Some claimants lost one or more relatives in the disaster and suffered 'pathological grief' or 'pathological mourning' which was also a psychiatric illness and meant grief the extent and duration of which was in excess of normal grief reaction.

That posed a difficult problem since a person was not to be compensated for normal grief but was to be compensated for pathological grief. Normal grief varied widely between one individual and another. The arbitrators had to estimate the extent to which each claimant's grief was in excess of the normal grief he or she would have suffered had the death occurred in ordinary circumstances and compensate the claimant accordingly. That was an enormously difficult task, which could only be done in a very rough and ready fashion, especially since in all these cases there was another form of illness present.

Some claimants continued to suffer to a significant extent, although in all cases improvement was probable. Although the victim would never forget the experience, and painful intrusive thoughts would never cease, the improvement would reach a point at which, despite remaining intrusive thoughts, the victim was no longer suffering from psychiatric illness.

Since compensation for nervous shock was compensation for psychiatric illness, it was the period until the illness ceased which was compensatable. That had had to be assessed, as was everything else, on a balance of probabilities, and for obvious reasons, the estimate approached a 'guestimate'. The prognoses were guarded in cases in which a claimant was still ill. The arbitrators also bore in mind that, very understandably, come claimants were reluctant to undergo treatment which involved recollecting the distressing circumstances of the disaster.

153

The awards also took account of the risk of future psychiatric troubles. An injury to a limb left it vulnerable to trouble at the slightest cause. It was the same with psychiatric problems. The claimants would be at risk of further illness in the face of stress which would not have affected them or would have affected them less but for their Zeebrugge experience. The reported cases contained no clear guidelines on damages for nervous shock, and the arbitrators' assessments were based upon how each claimant's illness compared with cases in which damages were awarded for physical injuries.

The awards ranged from £1,750 to £30,000.

Post Traumatic Stress Disorder versus Post Traumatic Stress Reaction

When I first started interviewing for this book there was one major pitfall I failed to recognise. It is the necessity to distinguish clearly between Post Traumatic Stress *Disorder* and Post Traumatic Stress *Reaction*. When I had finished talking to Pauline Chesterton it was clear that she was a victim of the former. I then wondered if her rapist, or any rapist for that matter, recognising what he had done and the damage he had caused, could suffer similarly. I interviewed one such man and came away thinking, yes, he does have the same problem. And I believe that in a broad sense he did. He certainly had many of the same symptoms. However, the more I interviewed the more I became aware of the difference between disorder and reaction, and this distinction is of particular importance if dealt with by the legal profession during a court case without having been clearly defined by the medical profession.

Let us suppose a man is on trial for murder. He has all the symptoms consistent with post traumatic stress. If it can be proved that he suffered from Post Traumatic Stress *Disorder* prior to the crime, his defence can legitimately advance this as a case of diminished responsibility at the time of the murder – as has frequently been done, successfully, in the United States. However, if the man is suffering from

155

Post Traumatic Stress *Reaction*, it could well be argued that he was in full possession of all his faculties at the time of the crime, and that the *reaction* was a result of the crime, not in any way the cause. It is a difficult problem for lawyers to work out, bearing in mind that the symptoms for both disorder and reaction are so difficult to separate, if at all. I excluded my interview with the rapist for this reason. I could not decide to my own satisfaction whether it was a case of disorder or reaction.